Second edition

Nursing Adults with Long Term Conditions

Jane Nicol

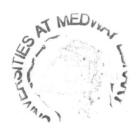

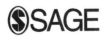 |

Los Angeles | London | New Delhi
Singapore | Washington DC

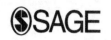

Learning Matters
An imprint of SAGE Publications Ltd
1 Oliver's Yard
55 City Road
London EC1Y 1SP

SAGE Publications Inc.
2455 Teller Road
Thousand Oaks, California 91320

SAGE Publications India Pvt Ltd
B 1/I 1 Mohan Cooperative Industrial Area
Mathura Road
New Delhi 110 044

SAGE Publications Asia-Pacific Pte Ltd
3 Church Street
#10-04 Samsung Hub
Singapore 049483

Editor: Alex Clabburn
Development editor: Richenda Milton-Daws
Production controller: Chris Marke
Project management: Swales & Willis Ltd,
Exeter, Devon
Marketing manager: Camille Richmond
Cover design: Wendy Scott
Typeset by: C&M Digitals (P) Ltd, Chennai, India
Printed in Great Britain by
CPI Group (UK) Ltd, Croydon, CR0 4YY

© Jane Nicol 2015

First published 2011
Second edition 2015

Library of Congress Control Number: 2015943493

British Library Cataloguing in Publication data

A catalogue record for this book is available from
the British Library

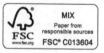

MIX
Paper from
responsible sources
FSC
www.fsc.org   FSC® C013604

ISBN 978-1-4739-1431-5
ISBN 978-1-4739-1432-2 (pbk)

At SAGE we take sustainability seriously. Most of our products are printed in the UK using FSC papers and boards.
When we print overseas we ensure sustainable papers are used as measured by the Egmont grading system.
We undertake an annual audit to monitor our sustainability.

Nursing Adults with Long Term Conditions

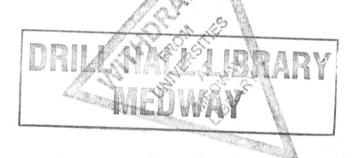

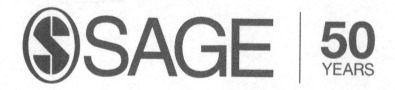

SAGE was founded in 1965 by Sara Miller McCune to support the dissemination of usable knowledge by publishing innovative and high-quality research and teaching content. Today, we publish more than 850 journals, including those of more than 300 learned societies, more than 800 new books per year, and a growing range of library products including archives, data, case studies, reports, and video. SAGE remains majority-owned by our founder, and after Sara's lifetime will become owned by a charitable trust that secures our continued independence.

Los Angeles | London | New Delhi | Singapore | Washington DC

This book is dedicated to:

Neil Anderson

Contents

Transforming Nursing Practice is a series tailor-made for pre-registration student nurses. Each book in the series is:

- Affordable
- Mapped to the NMC Standards and Essential Skills Clusters
- Full of active learning features
- Focused on applying theory to practice

Each book addresses a core topic and they have been carefully developed to be simple to use, quick to read and written in clear language.

> An invaluable series of books that explicitly relates to the NMC standards.
> Each book cover a different topic that students need to explore in order
> to develop into a qualified nurse... I would recommend this series to all
> Pre-Registration nursing students whatever their field or year of study.
>
> **Linda Robson**
> **Senior Lecturer, Edge Hill University**
>
> The set of books is an excellent resource for students. The series is small,
> easily portable and valuable. I use the whole set on a regular basis.
>
> **Fiona Davies**
> **Senior Nurse Lecturer, University of Derby**
>
> I recommend the SAGE/Learning Matters series to all my students
> as they are relevant and concise. Please keep up the good work.
>
> **Thomas Beary**
> **Senior Lecturer in Mental Health Nursing, University of Hertfordshire**

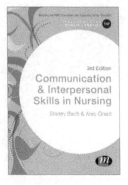

3rd Edition
Communication
& Interpersonal
Skills in Nursing
Shirley Bach & Alec Grant

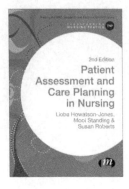

2nd Edition
Patient
Assessment and
Care Planning
in Nursing
Lioba Howatson-Jones,
Mooi Standing &
Susan Roberts

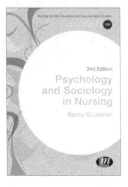

2nd Edition
Psychology
and Sociology
in Nursing
Benny Goodman

ABOUT THE SERIES EDITORS

Professor Shirley Bach is Head of the School of Health Sciences at the University of Brighton and responsible for the core knowledge titles. Previously she was head of post-graduate studies and has developed curriculum for undergraduate and pre-registration courses in a variety of subject domains.

Dr Mooi Standing is an Independent Academic Consultant (UK and International) and responsible for the personal and professional learning skills titles. She is an accredited NMC Quality Assurance Reviewer of educational programmes and a Professional Regulator Panellist on the NMC Practice Committee.

Sandra Walker is Senior Teaching Fellow in Mental Health at the University of Southampton and responsible for the mental health nursing titles. She is a Qualified Mental Health Nurse with a wide range of clinical experience spanning more than 20 years.

CORE KNOWLEDGE TITLES:

Becoming a Registered Nurse: Making the Transition to Practice
Communication and Interpersonal Skills in Nursing (3rd Ed)
Contexts of Contemporary Nursing (2nd Ed)
Getting into Nursing (2nd Ed)
Health Promotion and Public Health for Nursing Students (2nd Ed)
Introduction to Medicines Management in Nursing
Law and Professional Issues in Nursing (3rd Ed)
Leadership, Management and Team Working in Nursing (2nd Ed)
Learning Skills for Nursing Students
Medicines Management in Children's Nursing
Nursing and Collaborative Practice (2nd Ed)
Nursing and Mental Health Care
Nursing in Partnership with Patients and Carers
Passing Calculations Tests for Nursing Students (3rd Ed)
Palliative and End of Life Care in Nursing
Patient Assessment and Care Planning in Nursing (2nd Ed)
Patient and Carer Participation in Nursing
Patient Safety and Managing Risk in Nursing
Psychology and Sociology in Nursing (2nd Ed)
Successful Practice Learning for Nursing Students (2nd Ed)
Understanding Ethics for Nursing Students
Using Health Policy in Nursing
What is Nursing? Exploring Theory and Practice (3rd Ed)

PERSONAL AND PROFESSIONAL LEARNING SKILLS TITLES:

Clinical Judgement and Decision Making for Nursing Students (2nd Ed)
Critical Thinking and Writing for Nursing Students (2nd Ed)
Evidence-based Practice in Nursing (2nd Ed)
Information Skills for Nursing Students
Reflective Practice in Nursing (2nd Ed)
Succeeding in Essays, Exams & OSCEs for Nursing Students
Succeeding in Literature Reviews and Research Project Plans for Nursing Students (2nd Ed)
Successful Professional Portfolios for Nursing Students (2nd Ed)
Understanding Research for Nursing Students (2nd Ed)

MENTAL HEALTH NURSING TITLES:

Assessment and Decision Making in Mental Health Nursing
Engagement and Therapeutic Communication in Mental Health Nursing
Medicines Management in Mental Health Nursing
Mental Health Law in Nursing
Physical Healthcare and Promotion in Mental Health Nursing
Psychosocial Interventions in Mental Health Nursing

ADULT NURSING TITLES:

Acute and Critical Care in Adult Nursing (2nd Ed)
Caring for Older People in Nursing
Medicines Management in Adult Nursing
Nursing Adults with Long Term Conditions
Safeguarding Adults in Nursing Practice
Dementia Care in Nursing

You can find more information on each of these titles and our other learning resources at **www.sagepub.co.uk**. Many of these titles are also available in various e-book formats, please visit our website for more information.

About the author

Jane Nicol is a registered nurse and Senior Lecturer at the University of Worcester. During her career she has worked across a range of clinical settings in both primary and secondary care, enabling her to develop a broad knowledge and skill base. She currently teaches pre-registration nursing students, international nursing students, post-registration nurses and other healthcare professionals at the University of Worcester. Jane's main teaching focus is the care and management of people living with long term conditions and palliative and end of life care. Her particular areas of interest are interpersonal and intrapersonal skills, and the importance of these in allowing nurses to develop positive relationships with the people for whom they care.

Acknowledgements

The publishers and author would like to thank the following for their very helpful feedback during the writing of this book:

Maggie Roberts, Health Lecturer and Pathway Leader for Primary Care, and Chair of the Community Practice Learning Team, at the University of Nottingham;

Paul Macreth, Senior Lecturer and Course Leader for District Nursing, at Leeds Metropolitan University.

They would also like to thank Pilgrim Projects Ltd and the Patient Voices website (**www. patientvoices.org.uk**) for Bill's story and the accompanying word cloud (Figure 2.1) in the case study on page 29. The word cloud was created at **www.wordle.net**.

Introduction

About this book

People living with long term conditions (LTCs) are often experts in their own condition, living with and managing it on a day-to-day basis. Therefore, nurses and other healthcare professionals caring for, and working with, people living with LTCs have to possess the knowledge, skills and attributes that will foster partnership working, encourage self-management and support those whose condition requires more active care and management. The aim of this book is to provide an overview of the key aspects of the care and management of LTCs and to relate these to clinical practice. While the chapters in this book are presented sequentially, it is recognised that aspects of the care and management of a person living with an LTC, such as health promotion and symptom management, feature throughout their journey, from diagnosis through to palliative and end of life care. This book is primarily for adult nursing students; however it incorporates aspects of care from all fields of practice and is aimed at supporting the development of knowledge and skills across all fields of practice. Therefore this book may be of relevance and value for those studying child health, mental health and learning disability, as well as qualified health and social care professionals who are keen to develop their knowledge or who have mentoring roles.

A note on terminology

Given that the underlying premise of the care and management of long term conditions is based on self-care and self-management, the term 'person/individual' has been used, but when the context demands, the term 'patient' has been used.

Book structure

As mentioned previously, the chapters in this book are written sequentially and are designed to take you on the journey a person with an LTC travels from diagnosis through to palliative care. However, the book can be read by dipping in and out of chapters, though it is recommended that Chapter 1 is read first. Chapter 1 provides an overview of LTCs, their impact across the lifespan, and the importance of planning for transition of care from child to adult services. Models of care delivery and the impact LTCs have on individuals, both physically and psychologically, are explored.

In Chapter 2, the focus is on developing and maintaining effective therapeutic relationships with both the person living with an LTC and their carer. The concept of emotional intelligence is examined and its relevance to the therapeutic relationship discussed. The importance of effective communication is reviewed with some useful communication strategies outlined and related to LTCs. Chapter 3 uses an exploration of determinants of health and public health to set the context of health promotion in LTCs demonstrating the multifactorial nature of health and health promotion. The importance of health promotion in LTCs is explained and applied to practice; health promotion models are outlined and their relevance to LTCs discussed. Strategies for health promotion such as motivational interviewing are examined and related to people living with an LTC. Chapter 4 focuses on the importance of promoting self-management for people living with an LTC. It emphasises the importance of empowerment and how this can be promoted for people living with an LTC. By examining the skills and knowledge necessary to become successful self-managers, and by applying them to clinical scenarios, autonomy and empowerment of people living with LTCs can be increased. In Chapter 5, quality of life and symptom management in long term conditions are addressed, highlighting the areas of a person's life that influence and affect their quality of life. Effective symptom management is discussed using a framework such as the nursing process to support care. In Chapter 6, the emphasis is on case management. The roles and responsibilities of case managers are reflected upon, explored and related to case scenarios. Strategies to support complex care, such as care pathways and effective discharge planning, emphasise the need for collaborative working in the care and management of people living with an LTC.

Chapter 7 is the final chapter and introduces palliative care as a key part of the care and management of people with LTCs. The concept of 'bad news' is discussed and the importance of effective communication skills when breaking 'bad news' are emphasised and reflected upon. Specific strategies, including assessment frameworks, that can be used to support person-centred palliative and end of life care are examined and related to clinical practice.

Requirements for the NMC Standards for Pre-registration Nursing Education and the Essential Skills Clusters

The Nursing and Midwifery Council (NMC) has established standards of competence to be met by applicants to different parts of the register, and these are the standards it considers necessary for safe and effective practice. In addition to the competencies, the NMC has set out specific skills that nursing students must be able to perform at various points of an education programme. These are known as Essential Skills Clusters (ESCs). This book is structured so that it will help you to understand and meet the standards of competence and ESCs required for entry to the NMC register. The relevant competencies and ESCs are presented at the start of each chapter so that you can clearly see which ones the chapter addresses. There are *generic standards* that all nursing students irrespective of their field must achieve, and *field-specific standards* relating to each field of nursing – mental health, children's, learning disability and adult nursing. Most chapters use generic standards, but field-specific standards are occasionally presented as well.

Learning features

Throughout this book you will be presented with a range of learning activities that will help you to understand what you are reading. A series of case studies have been included to support the integration of theory and practice. These activities will encourage you to undertake some further independent study and to think more critically about the topics being discussed. Some of the activities will ask you to reflect on your previous clinical experience; reflection allows you to develop your understanding of yourself and your nursing practice and to identify how things can be improved. Where relevant, sample answers are provided at the end of each chapter; it is hoped that these activities will encourage you to become increasingly self-directed in your learning. It may be appropriate for you to consider completing these activities and including these in your personal and professional development portfolio.

Chapter 1
Long term conditions across the lifespan

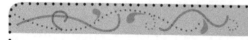

> Chapter aims
>
> After reading this chapter you will be able to:
>
> - describe the difference between an LTC and an acute condition;
> - discuss the incidence of LTCs and their impact on healthcare provision;
> - understand how the care and management of people living with a long term condition are organised;
> - reflect on the physical and psychological impacts of living with LTCs;
> - recognise the importance of appropriate care during the transition from child to adult services.

Introduction

You're looking over your shoulder the whole time, does he have his inhalers with him, do we have a spare one? Will he, or his friends know what to do if he has an attack . . .

(Mother of a 14-year-old boy living with asthma)

I wish I had listened to the advice that people gave me years ago. When you're younger you think 'it's not going to happen to me', ok, so my glucose level's a bit high so what! Now look at me, 47, in a wheelchair and I can't play with my kids.

(Male (47) diagnosed with type 1 diabetes at the age of 8)

It takes you a long time to readjust; I still think I can do everything I did before. I'm slowly learning that this is not the case, it's frustrating and it gets you down, but with support you can find a way.

(Female (45) following clipping of a cerebral aneurysm
after subarachnoid haemorrhage)

Diagnosis of a long term condition (LTC) can occur at all stages across the lifespan, resulting in different implications for the person, their future and for those caring for them. For a child, and their family, a diagnosis of asthma will mean a lifetime of adjustment and self-management of their condition. For a person diagnosed with type 1 diabetes it may mean making lifestyle choices that they do not want to make, or living with the consequences. For a person learning to live with the long term complications of a condition this could mean a long process of readjustment and finding new ways of doing things. Not only will their immediate concerns be different, the impact that their condition has on their day-to-day life will vary across the person's life. This will result in a range of needs having to be met, with the impact being felt physically, emotionally, socially and psychologically. In order for you to effectively support people living with LTCs, their family and carers, it is important to have an understanding of what LTCs are, their incidence across the lifespan and the frameworks used to guide their care and management. In order to do this, this chapter will develop your knowledge and understanding about LTCs, including transition of care from child to adult services and the importance of recognising the physical and psychological impact of living with LTCs.

Activity 1.1   *Critical thinking*

The Department of Health (DH) defines an LTC as: *a condition that cannot, at present, be cured but is controlled by medication and/or other treatment/therapies* (DH, 2013).

Using the above quote as a starting point, take some time to answer these questions.

- How many LTCs can you list?
- How do acute conditions and LTCs differ in relation to diagnosis, treatment, prognosis and outcome?

A brief outline answer is given at the end of the chapter.

Activity 1.1 has drawn your attention to the complex nature of LTCs, their varying signs and symptoms, care, management and prognosis. Over time it is likely that the symptoms of the condition become worse and there is a gradual, or sometimes sudden, deterioration in the health and wellbeing of the person living with the condition.

The incidence and impact of LTCs globally and in the UK

Globally LTCs account for over 36 million deaths each year, with most early deaths (those before the age of 60) occurring in low and middle income countries (WHO, 2013). In the UK, people in the lower socioeconomic groups have a 60% higher incidence of LTCs than those in the higher groups (DH, 2013). Globally cardiovascular disease, cancers, respiratory diseases and diabetes account for 80% of all deaths and between them they share the following risk factors: tobacco use, physical inactivity, harmful alcohol use and unhealthy diets (WHO, 2013). This highlights and emphasises the fact that the majority of LTCs are exacerbated by lifestyle choices.

Living with an LTC can have a profound effect on a person's quality of life. Over 40% of people living with one LTC and over 80% of people living with three or more report chronic pain (DH, 2013). However, the impact of LTCs can be felt beyond the person and their family. Globally the rise in LTCs, and the associated health costs in low income countries, can reduce household incomes; this in turn forces people in to poverty and prevents economic development (WHO, 2013).

Since the National Health Service was founded in 1948, both life expectancy and the incidence of LTCs have increased. The Office for National Statistics (ONS) states that, today, the life expectancy for men in the UK is 78 years and for women 82 (ONS, 2014). In addition figures identify that the population of the UK is getting older, with the number of people over the age of 85 doubling to 3.5 million in 25 years, equating to 5% of the population (ONS, 2011). These developments have led to in an increase in the incidence and prevalence of LTCs, especially some cancers, e.g., prostate, chronic kidney disease and diabetes (DH, 2012).

The DH estimates that the number of people living with LTCs will remain relatively stable over the next 10 years, but that the number of people living with multiple LTCs will rise from 1.9 million (in 2008) to 2.9 million in 2018 (DH, 2012). Figures from the DH (2012) estimate that approximately 10% of children under the age of 10 are living with one or more LTC, and of this 2% are living with a mental health LTC and 4% are living with asthma. By the age of 60, 40% of people have one or more LTCs, rising to 70% in the over 80s (DH, 2012).

The most common LTCs are diabetes, mental health problems, hypertension, asthma, musculoskeletal problems and heart disease (DH, 2012). In the UK people living with LTCs are the most intensive users of health and social care services, accounting for just over 50% of all general practitioner (GP) appointments and about 70% of all inpatient bed days (DH, 2013). Therefore, to promote well-being and to reduce pressures on health and social care services, the care and management for people with LTCs should focus on delaying the progression of LTCs through effective self-management. Combatting LTCs, both in the UK and globally, requires change on many levels, from supporting a person to make a change in their lifestyle to promoting public health policies that promote the prevention of LTCs.

Case study: Frazer

Frazer was diagnosed with type 1 diabetes when he was 8 years old. As a child Frazer was supported in managing his condition by his parents, however as he grew up and became a young person he did not manage his diabetes well. He started to smoke and drink heavily; this made it harder for him to maintain his blood glucose levels below 7.8 mmol/l and throughout his early adulthood his blood glucose levels were consistently raised.

Frazer lives with his partner Claire and their 11-year-old daughter Fiona. Claire works full time for a local whisky distillery. Frazer works part time as an office administrator and takes care of his daughter after school. Frazer stopped smoking 5 years ago; however he continues to drink alcohol on a daily basis, despite being asked to stop by family and healthcare professionals.

Frazer is now 47 years old and was diagnosed with diabetic **polyneuropathy** *in his late 30s; this means that he has reduced nerve sensation in his feet. He has had both great toes amputated as a result of this; in addition he has had longstanding problems with foot ulcers and recurrent infections. Most recently Frazer has received negative pressure wound therapy as an inpatient to try and prevent amputation of his lower leg.*

Activity 1.2   *Critical thinking*

Read the case study above, about Frazer, and answer the following questions.

- Over the course of his disease progression what health and social care services would Frazer and his family access?
- What impact will Frazer's LTC have on his family?

A brief outline answer is given at the end of the chapter.

Activity 1.2 emphasises the impact caring and managing LTCs has not only for health and social care services but for the family of the person living with the condition. Over the course of their life people living with LTCs will have contact with many health and social care professionals. Their care may be delivered in a **primary**, **secondary** or **tertiary** care setting. However, recent policy (NHS, Scotland 2010; Department of Health, Social Services and Public Safety (DHSSPS) 2012; NHS England, 2014; Wales Audit Office, 2014) emphasises the importance of health promotion and self-management in LTCs with out of hospital care playing a larger part in overall NHS services. This is reflected in Activity 1.2 where it can be seen that the majority of Frazer's care and management is provided in primary care. In all of these documents there is a clear emphasis on the importance of working with the person to provide patient-centred care, promote empowerment, self-care and management. As an LTC progresses, professionals are expected to deliver effective care and case management and prepare for palliative care requirements.

Quality Outcome Framework

The Quality Outcome Framework (QOF) is part of the General Medical Services (GMS) contract for GPs that was implemented in 2004. This points-based system rewards general practices for excellence in the following domains: clinical care, organisation, patient experience and additional services. Within the QOF the clinical care focuses on the successful management of the most common LTCs through the use of specific indicators (see Table 1.1).

Conditions listed on the QOF (listed alphabetically)	Examples of QOF indicators (listed alphabetically)
• Asthma • Atrial fibrillation • Cancer • Chronic kidney disease (CKD) • Chronic obstructive pulmonary disease • Coronary heart disease • Dementia	• Achieving target blood pressure, e.g. maintaining a blood pressure of 150/90 for people with hypertension • Achieving target cholesterol level • Confirming diagnosis with objective measures, e.g. echocardiogram confirming heart failure • Condition-specific reviews, e.g. retinal screening for people with diabetes

• Depression	• Influenza immunization, e.g. for those with COPD
• Diabetes mellitus	• Maintaining an accurate register of each condition – applicable to all LTCs
• Epilepsy	
• Heart failure	• Measuring blood pressure
• Hypertension	• Measuring cholesterol
• Hypothyroid	• Offering smoking cessation advice
• Learning disability	• Other condition-specific outcomes, e.g. lifestyle advice for people with cardiovascular disease
• Mental health	
• Obesity	• Recording person's smoking status
• Palliative care	• Specific therapy, e.g. lithium therapy for psychotic disorders
• Smoking	
• Stroke and transient ischaemic attack (TIA)	• Taking condition-specific blood tests, e.g. thyroid function tests for those with hypothyroid

Table 1.1: Quality Outcome Framework LTCs and examples of performance indicators (NHS Employers, 2014)

As you can see from Table 1.1, the QOF framework focuses on those LTCs with the greatest prevalence in the UK and incorporates areas of care such as health promotion, medication management and review to maximise efficacy. The aim of this is to improve patient prognosis, reduce disease burden and improve quality of life. You can find the latest advice on the QOF framework at **www.bma.org.uk/qofguidance**.

Models of care to support people living with one or more LTCs

Within the UK the theoretical frameworks that can be used to organise services and care in the management of LTCs focus on increasing the level of control and input a person living with an LTC has in relation to how services are delivered and in managing their condition. The main service delivery model that is reflected in all frameworks is the Kaiser Permanente service delivery model (see Figure 1.1). The Kaiser Permanente approach is underpinned by promoting health within the population as a whole, e.g. smoking cessation and healthy eating. For people with LTCs the approach includes self-care/support, disease/care management and case management.

Examples of strategies that can be used in each of the areas of the triangle in Figure 1.1 include:

• For supported self-care/management – action planning, health promotion and assistive technology.

• For disease/care management – personalised care planning, further support to enable self-management and access to specialist healthcare teams.

• For case management – integrated assessment and care planning and risk assessment.

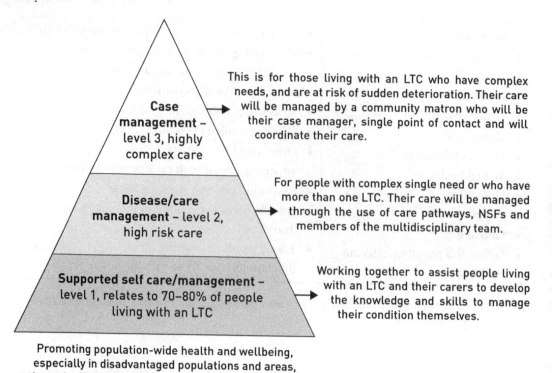

Case management – level 3, highly complex care → This is for those living with an LTC who have complex needs, and are at risk of sudden deterioration. Their care will be managed by a community matron who will be their case manager, single point of contact and will coordinate their care.

Disease/care management – level 2, high risk care → For people with complex single need or who have more than one LTC. Their care will be managed through the use of care pathways, NSFs and members of the multidisciplinary team.

Supported self care/management – level 1, relates to 70–80% of people living with an LTC → Working together to assist people living with an LTC and their carers to develop the knowledge and skills to manage their condition themselves.

Promoting population-wide health and wellbeing, especially in disadvantaged populations and areas, through effective health promotion and public health (DH, 2005)

Figure 1.1: The NHS and Social Care long term conditions model

(Source: The pyramid structure is taken fro.)

Activity 1.3   *Decision-making*

Read over the following case scenarios and decide which level of care on the Kaiser Permanente triangle best suits their current needs.

Sian

Sian Jones is a 20-year-old student who has been living with asthma since the age of 11 and has just started a Sports Science degree at university, moving away from home for the first time. Sian enjoys playing hockey and netball and plays for the university teams in both these sports. She is enjoying her studies and is taking full advantage of 'student life'; she lives in a shared house with four other students who are on the same course as her. Sian has noticed that she is becoming more breathless and is having to use her ventolin inhaler more frequently than when she was at home. She is worried about this as it is affecting her ability to play sport. After discussing this with her coach she decides to see the practice nurse at her GP surgery.

Linda

Linda is 78 years old; she lives alone in a one-bedroomed bungalow that she rents from the local council. Linda has one son, aged 53, who visits her twice a week.

Linda was diagnosed with heart failure in her 60s when she presented to her GP with occasional chest pain and breathlessness. Initially Linda put this down to anxiety about her job; she was working in the catering department at the local hospital. Following a series of investigations, physical examination, EEG, and BNP (brain natriuretic peptide) blood test Linda was diagnosed with heart failure and was prescribed a diuretic, an ACE inhibitor and a beta blocker.

Linda has been living with heart failure for the past 10 years and has tried to make some changes in her lifestyle. She has changed her diet, but still smokes (10 a day) and is reluctant to take much exercise; she does not like going out on her own as she is anxious that she may become unwell. This has led Linda to become isolated from her local community and she has recently begun to feel that she is a burden on her son.

Peter

Peter is 55 years old, married to Sarah (53) and they have three children (25, 22 and 18). Their oldest child (a son) is living and working abroad in France; their middle child (a daughter) is working in a local estate agent and their youngest child (another daughter) has just started at university studying to be a primary school teacher. Both daughters still live at home. Peter works as a freelance graphic designer; Sarah is a librarian at the local library.

Peter was diagnosed with Alzheimer's disease about a year ago. Initially his GP diagnosed depression and he was started on antidepressants; however Peter's symptoms became worse: coming home from an appointment he got lost and had to phone Sarah as he couldn't remember how to get home. Following this incident Peter and Sarah went to see his GP again, and it was then that he was referred on for a neurology outpatient appointment. At this appointment the Mini Mental State Exam was used, alongside taking Peter and Sarah's history and a physical examination, and a provisional diagnosis of Alzheimer's was made.

Following his diagnosis Peter was commenced on donepezil (Aricept) which he found improved his memory and his ability to find the right words. He has been able to carry on working, though he focuses on online consultancy (Sarah helps with the computer side of things) and works closer to home. Sarah has reduced the hours she works so that she can drive Peter to his appointments as he still struggles with directions.

A brief outline answer is given at the end of the chapter.

During the course of their disease progression people living with LTCs will move from one part of the triangle to another. As you can see from Activity 1.3, Linda is currently in the disease/ care management section. However, should she become more symptomatic and her health deteriorates, it may be that she progresses to the case management section of the triangle. People living with LTCs can also move up and down the triangle. For example, following a relapse of her asthma Sian may access specific disease management; then, once she has recovered from this she would return to supported self-care/management. This model of service delivery can be applied to any person living with any LTC.

The requirement to have a more integrated model that is proactive, holistic and preventative has led to the development of the House of Care (Coulter et al., 2013). This is one aspect of a range of programmes focused on strategies to ensure that all people living with LTCs have access to collaborative care planning and effective self-management support. It is about a whole systems approach that places the person living with the LTC at the heart of the delivery of care. Their care is driven and supported by effective commissioning and organisation of services and health and social care professionals who are committed to partnership working.

The impact of living with an LTC

As the quotations at the start of this chapter indicate, a diagnosis of an LTC can have a negative impact on the person and their family. Such a diagnosis is generally seen as being 'bad news', that is to say, news that implies the loss of something. The loss can relate to physical ability, loss of mobility due to motor neurone disease, something/someone that an individual values, altered body image (e.g. following mastectomy) which affects the way in which a person sees themselves, or loss of position in the family. The diagnosis of an LTC is usually given by a member of the medical profession. However, as a member of the healthcare team involved in that person's care, it is important that you are aware of the information a person has the right to know at the time of their diagnosis. The General Medical Council in their Good Medical Practice Guide (2013) states that a person has the right to know: their diagnosis, likely progression, treatment options, the outcome of treatment, side-effects of any treatment and the cost of the treatment options where relevant. During this initial consultation it is unlikely that the person will hear all that is being said and will leave with questions to ask. Adler et al. (1989) recognise the impact of physical and psychological noise on communication: physical noise could include the environment that the interaction is taking place in and sensory impairment, and psychological noise could be the distractions, fears and preconceptions, of both the patient and the nurse, that are brought to the situation.

Case study: Angela

Following the birth of her son Charlie six months ago, Angela (aged 28) has been feeling tired and has been experiencing muscular aches and pains. Initially she put these down to being a 'new mum'; however she was persuaded to see her general practitioner (GP) by her husband James. She has been undergoing a series of investigations and she is attending an appointment with her consultant to find out the results of the investigations. Both James and Charlie have come along to the appointment with Angela.

> You are on placement in the outpatient department, and the consultant has asked that your mentor sits in on Angela's consultation – you go in with her. It is during this consultation that Angela is given her diagnosis of relapsing remitting multiple sclerosis (RRMS).

Activity 1.4   *Critical thinking*

Read Angela's case study above, and answer the following questions. You may want to discuss your thoughts with a fellow student and compare notes.

- What physical and psychological noise may impact on Angela and James's ability to take on board information?
- What could you do to minimise the impact of these?

A brief outline answer is given at the end of the chapter.

Activity 1.4 demonstrates the need for ongoing communication for people diagnosed with LTCs and their family. You should provide relevant information in an appropriate format and recap as necessary to ensure that the information has been understood by the person and their family. The impact of living with LTCs goes beyond the point of diagnosis and stays with the person and their family as their condition progresses. It is important therefore to remember that 'noise' may be present at other times during a person's health journey. People living with LTCs will feel the impact of their diagnosis in all areas of their life, physically, psychologically and socially. The remainder of this section will discuss the physical and psychological impact of living with LTCs. The social impact will be discussed in Chapter 3 in relation to **determinants of health** and public health.

The physical impact of living with an LTC

Many of the physical effects of living with LTCs are condition-specific. There is not scope in this section to outline the altered pathology and the signs and symptoms of all LTCs; therefore the remainder of this section will outline the altered physiology and the main signs and symptoms of the following LTCs: asthma, chronic heart failure, epilepsy, prostate cancer, HIV and dementia. Information on the altered physiology and the signs and symptoms of coronary heart disease, rheumatoid arthritis and Parkinson's disease can be found in Activity 5.1 in Chapter 5.

Asthma

Asthma is an inflammatory lung condition where the airways in the lungs are hyper-responsive to a range of irritants. Asthma can be described as being intrinsic, where no specific irritant can be found, or extrinsic, where an identifiable irritant is present. Such irritants include smoke, pollen, household allergens (e.g. dust mites), medication (e.g. non-steroidal anti-inflammatory drugs) and infection (e.g. upper respiratory tract). When exposed to an irritant, the muscle in the airways contracts, and the membranes shrink, resulting in a narrowing of the airways. As the airway narrows, the flow of air to the lungs is disrupted, resulting in an 'asthma attack' where the person experiences wheeze, chest tightness, shortness of breath and coughing (Clinical Knowledge Summaries (CKS), 2013). As well as narrowing of the airways the irritants cause inflammation of the membranes and excessive production of mucus (Lorig et al., 2006). This inflammatory response is reversible; however, if it is not managed correctly it can lead to complication such as respiratory failure, **status asthmaticus** and irreversible damage of the airways. Asthma can also lead to fatigue, resulting in time off work or school (CKS, 2013).

Chronic heart failure

Chronic heart failure (CHF) can be associated with previous myocardial infarction or other cardiovascular conditions, e.g. hypertension. It can be caused by either high or low cardiac output. High cardiac output is where the heart is working at a normal or increased rate but the requirements of the body are more than the heart can supply, e.g. anaemia, hyperthyroidism. Low cardiac output is caused by a reduction in the function of the heart and is due to the following (Simon et al., 2014):

- increased pre-loading of the heart, e.g. fluid overload or mitral regurgitation;
- failure of the pumping mechanism of the heart, e.g. ischaemic heart disease;
- inadequate heart rate, e.g. use of beta blockers;
- arrhythmia, e.g. atrial fibrillation;
- excessive overloading, e.g. hypertension.

When discussing CHF it is common to use the terms 'right heart failure' and 'left heart failure', resulting in differing signs and symptoms due to the nature of the heart failure. Right heart failure is usually associated with congestion of the veins throughout the person's body while left heart failure is usually associated with congestion of the pulmonary veins (CKS, 2014a). In right heart failure a person can experience the following: ankle oedema, abdominal discomfort due to liver distension, fatigue and nausea and anorexia. People with left heart failure can experience the following: shortness of breath (on exertion) and **orthopnea**, fatigue, reduced exercise tolerance and nocturnal cough (Simon et al., 2014; CKS, 2014a).

Epilepsy

Epilepsy is a neurological condition that is caused by abnormal bursts of electrical activity in the brain due to increased neural activity. This presents as a **transient** disturbance of consciousness, behaviour, emotion, motor function or sensation (CKS, 2014b). These episodes are called epileptic seizures and can last from a few seconds to a few minutes. Epilepsy is not a single condition; therefore the symptoms occurring during a seizure will vary depending on the part of the brain affected by the increase in neural activity (Drennan and Goodman, 2014).

- Focal epilepsy – this involves one part of the body; seizures will start in that part and then progress to other parts of the body, becoming generalised (Jacksonian epilepsy).

- Grand mal epilepsy – this presents as a generalised seizure with sudden onset of **tonic** contraction of the muscles and **clonic** convulsions occurring on both sides of the body and at the same time. Following the seizure the person is usually unconscious and takes time to recover.

- Petit mal epilepsy – this is characterised by a pause in speech or activity, with the person being unaware of the episode.

- Myoclonic epilepsy – this is a variation of petit mal epilepsy, resulting in **atonic** drop attacks.

- Temporal lobe epilepsy – during seizures the person may remain conscious and can experience sensory, emotional and cognitive changes, including oral and auditory hallucinations.

Status epilepticus is a complication of epilepsy and occurs when a seizure lasts more than 30 minutes, or a person has successive convulsions where they do not recover consciousness between the seizures (CKS, 2014b). Treatment aims to stop seizures from occurring; however, should this not be possible the aim is to reduce their frequency and severity. Epilepsy can have a significant impact on the day-to-day life of a person; it may affect their work, education and leisure activities (CKS, 2014b). Therefore providing information regarding epilepsy, the day-to-day management and how to manage seizures increases a person's sense of control and minimises the stigma attached to the condition.

Prostate cancer

Prostate cancer is the most common cancer in men: more than 34,000 men are diagnosed with prostate cancer each year (Cancer Research UK, 2010). The prostate gland is found only in men; it lies just beneath the bladder and is normally the size of a walnut and is divided into two lobes. The urethra runs through the middle of the prostate: the main function of the prostate is to produce fluid which enriches and protects sperm. The growth and function of the prostate gland depends on the production of testosterone, a hormone produced in the testes. Prostate cancer develops due to the formation of abnormal cells in the prostate gland. These cells cause the prostate to increase in size: as prostate cancer is a slow-growing cancer, in the early stages of the disease there may be no symptoms. Symptoms of local prostate cancer include urinary retention and haematuria; frequency of micturition and urgency can be present. As the cancer spreads the person may experience symptoms such as weight loss, bone pain and fatigue (Simon et al., 2014).

Human immunodeficiency virus (HIV)

HIV is a retrovirus that causes infections; the long term symptoms of the condition and the condition itself develop slowly over a period of time. Two species of HIV have been identified: HIV-1, which is highly contagious and transmittable and is found throughout the world; and HIV-2, which is less contagious and transmittable and is predominately found in West Africa and Portugal (CKS, 2010a). HIV affects a person's immune system: HIV infects cells in the immune system, predominately CD4 cells. These cells are called t-helper cells and are crucial to activating cell immunity. The virus binds itself to the CD4 receptor and infects the CD4 cell with its ribonucleic acid (RNA). Due to its specific properties RNA is able to convert the viral RNA into DNA, which is then incorporated into the person's DNA. The virus then lies dormant until the CD4 cells are activated due to infection. When this occurs, new HIV enzymes are produced; these mature viruses then detach from the walls of the CD4 cell, enter the blood stream and infect other cells in the body (CKS, 2010a). In HIV the virus is present in all cell-containing body fluid, e.g. blood, semen, vaginal secretions, breast milk, pleural effusions and cerebrospinal fluid. Therefore transmission can occur when infected body fluid enters another person's blood stream, e.g. needle-stick injury and sexual activity. HIV leaves a person susceptible to infection, resulting in tiredness, pyrexia, and joint and muscle pain. Some of these symptoms can be mild and mistaken for other conditions, such as the common cold. HIV can progress into acquired immune deficiency syndrome (AIDS). Diagnosis is made on the basis of a low CD4 count, below 200, and if an AIDS-defining clinical condition is present, e.g. Kaposi's sarcoma, recurrent pneumonia or ongoing herpes simplex infection for more than one month (CKS, 2010a). At this point, due to the damage to the immune system, a person may be experiencing night sweats, weight loss, shortness of breath and pyrexia. Specialist support will be able to address the wide range of psychological, emotional, social and physical needs a person living with HIV may have.

Dementia

Dementia is a **syndrome** that occurs due to damage to a person's brain, resulting in many problems, such as memory loss, although their level of consciousness is not affected (Simon et al., 2014). Most of these syndromes progress gradually over a period of years; a person's ability to manage their activities of daily living (ADL) independently is affected by their declining memory and cognitive ability.

The symptoms of dementia occur in three areas (CKS, 2015):

1. Cognitive dysfunction – this results in a person experiencing many problems, e.g. language (both speech and written), memory and orientation to time, place and person.
2. Psychiatric and behavioural problems – these include personality changes, reduced emotional control (emotionally labile) and agitation.
3. Difficulties with ADLs – areas that are affected include driving, personal care and shopping.

The incidence of dementia in the population increases with age; conventionally a person developing dementia under the age of 65 is classed as having early or young-onset dementia. The most common causes of dementia are listed below (CKS, 2015).

- Alzheimer's disease accounts for approximately 50% of all cases of dementia. It is caused by degenerative changes in the cerebral cortex, resulting in pathological changes to the structure and chemistry of a person's brain. The cortex of the brain atrophies, and amyloid (fibrous protein) plaques form on and around the neurones. Neurones affected by this have reduced production of acetylcholine (a neurotransmitter involved in learning, memory and mood). Initially a person experiences memory lapses, e.g. forgetting names and places. As the disease progresses, symptoms like problems with language and mood changes (depression and agitation) occur.

- Vascular dementia accounts for about 25% of dementia cases and is sometimes called vascular cognitive impairment. Damage to the brain is as a result of cerebrovascular disease, including cerebrovascular accident (CVA), small undetected CVAs (multi-infarct) or ongoing changes in the small cerebral blood vessels (subcortical dementia). In this type of dementia each cerebrovascular event causes an increase in the person's symptoms; these include personality changes, some focal neurological deficit and apathy.

Management of dementia includes providing the person and their carer with strategies to manage their memory loss, social and carer support and management of presenting symptoms, e.g. agitation, sleep disturbance (Simon et al., 2014).

Activity 1.5 — *Evidence-based practice and research*

To further develop your understanding of the pathophysiology of LTCs, briefly outline the altered physiology and the main signs and symptoms of:

- RRMS;
- COPD;
- Type 1 diabetes.

Some useful resources:

- your preferred applied anatomy and physiology text books;
- **http://cks.nice.org.uk/#?char=A** – this is a useful website for healthcare professionals working in primary care, and provides evidence-based information on managing common conditions seen in primary care;
- **www.nhs.uk/Pages/HomePage.aspx** – this comprehensive website contains information on many health conditions.

A brief outline answer is given at the end of the chapter.

Activity 1.5 demonstrates the profound effect that the physical symptoms of LTCs can have on the day-to-day life of the person. Many of these, such as pain and fatigue, can be mentally exhausting to live with and can have a negative psychological impact on the person's mental wellbeing. Depression is known to occur in approximately 20% of people who are living with an LTC (NICE, 2009a).

The psychological impact of living with an LTC

People living with a condition such as type 2 diabetes, hypertension, CVA, COPD or end-stage renal disease are two to three times more likely to develop depression than people who are in good physical health (Haddad, 2010). It is known that living with LTCs can both cause and increase a person's depression. This **comorbidity** adversely affects the course and outcome of both their underlying LTC and their overlying mental health condition. Indeed, as the population ages and the incidence of LTCs increases for some people they will be faced with **multimorbidity**. For example, a person living with rheumatoid arthritis and type 2 diabetes, who is experiencing pain and reduced ability to manage their medication, has an increased risk of developing depression, which may, in turn, increase their pain and distress, creating a cycle of symptoms (NICE, 2009a). There is also evidence to suggest that depression can increase the likelihood of a person developing conditions such as heart disease (Nicholson et al., 2006) or type 2 diabetes (Mezuk et al., 2008). This is thought to be multifactorial; for example a sedentary lifestyle and poor diet (risk factors for heart disease) may be related to symptoms of depression, low energy levels, reduced motivation and lack of interest in day-to-day activities. Treatment side effects may increase the likelihood of a person developing depression, for example corticosteroids; this could be due to the fact that corticosteriods reduce serotonin levels. Additionally antidepressant medication is associated with an increase in a person's weight (Kivimäki et al., 2010), which if not managed could increase the person's chance of developing type 2 diabetes (Kivimäki et al., 2010). It is known that depression has a negative effect on a person's health outcome, their level of disability and how well they utilise available resources (Haddad, 2010). Given this complex interaction and the potential negative effect, diagnosing and managing depression is an important part of your care of those living with LTCs.

A formal diagnosis of depression is made using either the ICD-10 classification system or the DSM-IV system, with symptoms having been present for at least two weeks and evident on most days. When using these systems there are some key symptoms that need to be present for a diagnosis of depression to be made. These are: low mood, loss of interest and pleasure or loss of energy (NICE, 2009b). However, for people living with LTCs identifying depression can be challenging as many of the physical symptoms of depression (e.g. fatigue, insomnia and reduced appetite) may also be related to the LTC and its treatment. Therefore, it is important that you are alert to the possibility of a person developing depression. Although you will not be involved in diagnosing depression, your knowledge and understanding of an individual may alert you to changes in their mood that could indicate depression. NICE (2009a) recommends the Two-Question Screen Tool for people with LTCs who may have depression:

- During the last month, have you often been bothered by feeling down, depressed or hopeless?
- During recent months, have you often been bothered by having little interest or pleasure in doing things?

As these questions link to the key symptoms required for a diagnosis of depression to be made, this screening tool has excellent sensitivity (Haddad, 2010). If a person answers yes to one or both questions a more detailed assessment for depression should be undertaken. In situations where communication is difficult, e.g. sensory impairment or learning disability, a visual analogue like the distress thermometer can be used (NICE, 2009a). Using a picture of a thermometer and a scale of 0 to 10 it uses a single question screen: *How distressed have you been during the past week on a scale of 0 to 10?* If any significant level of distress is identified, a score of 4 or more, this should be reported and investigated further. If necessary a referral to specialist services, e.g. community learning disability services, should be made. Once a diagnosis of depression has been made, appropriate treatment and management is required. NICE (2009a) recommend the use of the stepped care framework, as outlined in Table 1.2.

Focus of the intervention	Nature of the intervention	Place of care
Step 4: Severe and complex depression, risk to life, severe self-neglect	Multiprofessional inpatient care, medication, high intensity psychological interventions	Specialist mental health in patient services
Step 3: Moderate to severe depression, persistent symptoms, poor response to treatment	Collaborative care, further assessment, combined treatments (medication/ psychological interventions)	Primary care, general hospital setting, access to specialist mental health services
Step 2: Mild to moderate depression, persistent symptoms	Low intensity psychosocial and psychological interventions, medication, further assessment and active monitoring	Primary care, general hospital setting, self-management
Step 1: All known or suspected presentations of depression	Assessment, monitoring, support, psycho-education and referral for further assessment	Primary care, self-care and self-management

Table 1.2: Stepped care for depression in LTCs

(Source: NICE, 2009a)

Activity 1.6 — *Reflection*

Reflecting back on your recent clinical experience, can you identify a situation where it would have been appropriate to ask the questions in the Two-Question Screen Tool described above?

If these questions had been asked would the person's response to these have altered your care? If so, how?

As the answers will be based on your own observations there is no outline answer at the end of this chapter.

Many people find discussing mental health issues uncomfortable; this applies to the person with the LTC and the healthcare professionals involved in their care. Activity 1.6 will have highlighted that in some cases addressing mental health issues relies on you having the confidence to discuss mental health issues with those in your care. The information in Chapter 2 of this book can be used to support you to develop effective therapeutic relationships, fostering a relationship that is open and non-judgemental. Developing trust in this way encourages those in your care to communicate their hopes and fears and can assist you in recognising changes in a person's mental health.

Care across the lifespan: the transition from child to adult services

As mentioned at the start of this chapter it is estimated that up to 10% of children under the age of 10 are living with LTCs (DH, 2012). Many of these children are living into adulthood and require continuing support and care during their adult years to enable them to successfully manage their condition in order to live as healthy and as independent a life as possible. It is important therefore that you gain an understanding of the role of transition within the care and management of children living with LTCs. This will enable you to work with child health professionals and better support those in your care. Adolescence is a time of change for all young people, with many social and psychological changes taking place, peer pressure, pushing boundaries and increasing responsibilities. However, young people living with LTCs face particular challenges. Young people need age-appropriate services that are responsive to their changing needs as they grow into adulthood. The DH describe transition as a process and not as an event and should be planned for early:

> *A purposeful, planned process that addresses the medical, psychosocial and educational/vocational needs of adolescents and young adults with chronic physical and medical conditions as they move from child-centred to adult-orientated health care system.*

> (DH, 2006, p. 14)

Transition should, at its heart, promote the autonomy, independence and aspirations of young people as they become young adults. This can be achieved if you place the young person at the centre of their transition being supported by collaborative care and management between health, social care and education. However, this is made difficult by the fact that some services stop at age 16, others at 18 and some will see young people past the age of 18 (CQC, 2014). It is known that organised transition programmes benefit young people and their families in many ways: improved follow-up, better disease control and improved documentation, resulting in improved communication and care. There is also evidence to suggest that poor transition and a lack of follow-up leads a young person to disengage from health services, and this can have a negative impact on their health (DH, 2008c). A report by New Philanthropy Capital (McGrath and Yeowart, 2009) noted that many of the needs of young people during transition were not being met by healthcare services but were being met by charities instead. Within the UK the charity Contact a Family (www.cafamily.org.uk) provides region-based information for families where a child has an LTC:

- *Preparing for adult life and transition: information for families, England and Wales;*
- *Preparing for adult life and transition – Northern Ireland;*
- *Preparing for adult life and transition – Scotland.*

The DH (2008c) recommends that transition from child to adult services should begin when a child is approximately 13 years old and support should continue until they are 25 years old. This is to tie in with an age when young people are already receiving advice regarding education and career choices. This approach allows the young person to plan their healthcare transition along-side planning for their future career and independence. However a 2014 report by the Care Quality Commission (CQC) identified that there is still work to be done. The Commission's findings indicated the following:

- Information about what changes to expect when they move to adult services was inconsistent.
- The process of transition was not well understood by young people, their families or some professionals delivering the care.
- Where guidance or protocols were in place they were not always used.
- Young people and their families say the system feels fragmented with parents indicating that they were the main coordinator of care; this was supported by care professionals.
- The transition process has rarely begun by the age of 14.

The CQC recommends that existing practice guidelines should be followed, including the use of health transition plans and health passports. They also state that there should be more involvement from GPs, especially in the planning stages for transition. Finally they recommend that there should be a change across the health service that recognises the specific needs of young people/adults.

Health transition plans

Working with appropriate members of the healthcare team, health transition plans are developed by the young person and focus on what they can do to stay healthy, minimise their health need and maximise their independence. This collaborative approach allows the young person to identify their needs and work with healthcare professionals to write up an action plan to meet these needs. By engaging the young person in the early stages there is the opportunity to increase their feelings of control and empowerment and to develop their self-management skills (DH, 2008c). A health transition plan should:

- assist the young person to become more knowledgeable and confident in making decisions that impact on their health and healthcare needs, e.g. action planning and self-management;
- support the young person in understanding their LTC and how to minimise the impact of their LTC on their future health and wellbeing, e.g. health education and health promotion;
- promote the sharing of information, where appropriate, between relevant health and social care services, e.g. health records being held by the young person;
- address transition in the context of the young person's life, taking into account all the person's needs, e.g. education.

In addition the health transition plan should focus on the young person's strengths and include all areas of the person's life. There should be a clear focus on promoting health and wellbeing and what is required to achieve this. The young person's physical, emotional (including sexual health) and social health should be assessed along with their ability for self-care, including any aids and adaptations required. The young person's ability to participate in the medical management of their LTC should also be assessed, including administration of medication. In the broader context of the young person's life their education, training and leisure requirements should also be assessed, with the aim being to maximise the young person's independence (DH, 2008c).

Health passports/action plans

These are documents that are held by the young person and their family and incorporate information about their LTC, medication and treatment, who is involved in their care and what is important to them. Its aim is to ensure that all relevant information about a young person's health and care requirements are kept in one place. It is designed to be a 'live' document and to be updated as the young person's circumstances change. It is not a clinical record; however it does ensure that relevant professionals have access to essential information about the young person, reducing the need for the young person and/or their family to repeat their health needs to different health teams (CQC, 2014).

For the parents of a young person the transition of care from child to adult health services can often cause anxiety. This is in part due to the increasing independence of the young person, who may now be making their own decisions, resulting in the parent feeling excluded (Allen et al., 2011). It is important therefore that transition planning incorporates not just the needs of the young person but the needs of the whole family. If the young person and their family work effectively with child health services early in the transition process, this will enable the young person to develop the required knowledge and skills to successfully manage their LTC into their adult life and will support the family in their changing roles.

Activity 1.7   *Reflection*

Reflecting back on your recent clinical experience and considering the information above, consider the following:

* What is your experience of how care has been provided and managed for young people?
* What were some of the challenges faced by both the young adult and their family?
* How might you have used a health transition plan/health passport to enhance their care?

As the answers will be based on your own observations there is no outline answer at the end of this chapter.

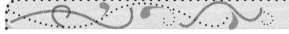

Chapter summary

This chapter has provided you with an overview of the impact of LTCs across the lifespan. It has outlined the incidence of LTCs in both adults and children and the impact this has on healthcare services and their design. In outlining the physical and psychological impact of living with LTCs it has identified the importance of having a good understanding of the signs and symptoms of a variety of LTCs. It has emphasised the need for timely and focused transition planning to ensure young people do not disengage from healthcare services at an important time in their health journey.

Having read this chapter and worked through the activities you will have developed your knowledge and skills in relation to the impact of LTCs across the lifespan. How you use this new knowledge will depend on where you are working and your roles and responsibilities. By increasing your understanding of how the care and management of LTCs is delivered, you will be able to liaise with other members of the healthcare team to provide an appropriate level of care. You can better support people living with LTCs by developing your knowledge and understanding of the physical and psychological impact of living with a variety of LTCs. This will enable you to provide care that directly meets the needs of the person and will enable you to plan appropriate care for future needs. By working with your child health colleagues you will be able to support young people during a crucial time in their healthcare journey, ensuring that they gain the necessary knowledge and skills to manage their LTC into adulthood.

Activities: brief outline answers

Activity 1.1 Critical thinking (page 6)

Some LTCs: asthma, arthritis (osteo and rheumatoid), diabetes (types 1 and 2), epilepsy, some cancers (prostate), chronic obstructive pulmonary disease (COPD), motor neurone disease (MND), cerebrovascular accident (CVA), dementia, depression, psoriasis, coronary heart disease (CHD), human immunodeficiency virus (HIV), Parkinson's disease, muscular dystrophy, hepatitis (B, C and D), chronic kidney disease, Crohn's disease, diverticulitis, cerebral palsy, cystic fibrosis, traumatic head injury, sensory impairment, e.g. deafness.

	Acute conditions	LTCs
Onset	Abrupt, for example, appendicitis, meningitis, pneumonia	Generally gradually over a period of time, though some conditions can progress rapidly, e.g. motor neurone disease
Duration	Limited duration, once over the initial episode. Though may result in some long term implication, e.g. cognitive impairment following meningitis	Present over a long period of time, with no definite end point

(Continued)

(Continued)

	Acute conditions	**LTCs**
Cause	Usually has a single cause, e.g. bacterial infection	May be due to lifestyle factors, genetics or cause may not be known. One LTC may result in other symptoms, e.g. type 1 diabetes may result in peripheral neuropathy
Diagnosis and prognosis	A diagnosis is usually made quickly and accurately	Diagnosis can take time, difficult to predict the outcome, can lead to uncertainty
Therapeutic interventions	Usually effective in managing the condition, e.g. targeted use of antibiotics for bacterial infection	Often only able to manage symptoms, side-effects present, e.g. triple therapy for HIV can cause fatigue and gastrointestinal upset
Outcome	Cure is possible	No cure is available

Activity 1.2 Critical thinking (page 8)

Over the course of his life it is likely that Frazer and his family will have come into contact with the following health and social care professionals and services.

- Primary healthcare team (PHCT): GP and practice nurse for ongoing monitoring of his type 1 diabetes involving regular blood tests, weight and blood pressure monitoring, health promotion regarding smoking and alcohol consumption and wound care. Support from the specialist community diabetes team regarding self-management of his type 1 diabetes and wound management. Access to community pharmacy for medication for regular medication prescriptions, and for advice regarding taking over the counter medication. Input from the community podiatry/chiropody team regarding foot health, correct foot wear and management of his ulcers.
- Secondary care services: regular review by outpatient services, both consultant and nurse specialist. In patient care for any severe foot ulcer infections and for negative pressure wound therapy and associated follow-up care.

This does not include access to services as a result of an emergency or for aspects of care not related to his type 1 diabetes.

Frazer's condition may affect his family in the following ways:

- Changing of roles and responsibilities within the family, both for Claire and Fiona, who may take on caring roles and responsibilities.
- Impact of Frazer's condition on Fiona, hospital and GP visits, not being able to play with her dad, not being as active.
- Making changes to the house to accommodate equipment that Frazer needs, e.g., wheelchair.
- Financial implications, cost of any adaptations, reduction in family income if Frazer is not able to work.
- Increase in stress for all family members, including the realisation that Frazer may become increasing less able as a result of his disease.

Activity 1.3 Decision-making (page 10)

Sian – supported self-care/management and disease/care management; Linda – disease/care management; Peter – supported self-care/management.

Activity 1.4 Critical thinking (page 13)

Physical noise
- There may be noise coming in from outside the room.
- Charlie may be crying/babbling.

Psychological noise

- They may be distracted by Charlie.
- They may have heard the words 'multiple sclerosis' and not listened to anything after that.
- They may be worried about each other.

Minimise physical noise

- Minimise disturbances, ensure phones are redirected, ask other staff to keep the area quiet.
- Offer to take Charlie out of the room while they are having their consultation.

Minimise psychological noise

- Spend some time ensuring Charlie is happy and settled, offer to take Charlie out of the room for the remainder of the consultation.
- Observe their verbal and non-verbal communication for signs of confusion and distress. Note at what point in the consultation this was at – it may be necessary to go over information later. Listen to their questions/comments – they will provide you with useful information as to how much they have heard/ understood and what may need to be recapped on.

Activity 1.5 Evidence-based practice and research (page 17)

RRMS

This is the most common type of multiple sclerosis (MS) and is characterised by numerous relapses and remissions. Relapses are periods of time where symptoms are worse; these are often followed by periods of remission where symptoms disappear or improve. Relapses may last for days, weeks or even months. During a relapse a person may experience new symptoms or may have a recurrence of previous symptoms (Drennan and Goodman, 2014).

MS is a neurological condition affecting a person's central nervous system (CNS). Nerve fibres in the CNS are surrounded and protected by myelin; this substance insulates the nerve fibres, allowing messages to travel quickly and smoothly within the CNS.

MS is an autoimmune condition: a person's body mistakes part of their own body as a foreign body and attacks it. In the case of MS it is the myelin that is attacked and damaged. This damage causes demyelination, where the myelin covering the nerve fibres is reduced and scars called lesions develop. Demyelination disrupts the messages travelling along the nerve fibres, e.g. slowing them down.

The symptoms of MS depend on the part of the CNS affected, but can include fatigue, continence problems, visual disturbances, muscle spasm and pain, and emotional problems such as depression (Drennan and Goodman, 2014). Depression is common in people with MS; it is present in as many as 29% of all cases.

COPD

This is a lung condition that is characterised by airflow obstruction; this is usually progressive with the obstruction being due to a combination of airway diseases, chronic bronchitis and emphysema. It is associated with an abnormal inflammatory response of the lungs to noxious stimuli, e.g. cigarette smoke (Drennan and Goodman, 2014).

Chronic bronchitis is clinically defined as a persistent cough with sputum production for at least three months of the year for two consecutive years. Cigarette smoke causes **hyperplasia** and **hypertrophy** of the mucus-secreting glands found in the large airways, e.g. bronchioles. As a result of this a person's small airways become obstructed with mucus plugs and oedema, resulting in a reduction of the action of the cilia, preventing the movement of mucus from the small to large airways to be expectorated. This reduces the level of gaseous exchange in the lungs.

Emphysema is the permanent enlargement of the air space **distal** to the terminal bronchiole as a result of alveolar septal destruction. As distal airways are held open by the alveolar septa this destruction causes the airways to collapse, resulting in obstruction. As the alveolar walls are destroyed, **bullae** form, and destruction of the parenchyma (gas exchange tissue) leads to a reduction in perfusion of oxygen from the lungs to the blood stream (Hickin et al., 2013). A person with COPD may present with breathlessness on exertion, chronic cough, frequent infections, fatigue and weight loss.

Type 1 diabetes

This condition occurs when a person's body does not produce insulin and often develops in teenage years and almost always before the age of 40. Insulin is a hormone produced by the pancreas: in type 1 diabetes autoimmune responses damage the beta cells of the islet cells in the pancreas. This results in a lack of insulin or no insulin being produced (Simon et al., 2014). Normally insulin is secreted by the pancreas as the level of glucose in the blood stream increases, usually associated with digestion of food, and is responsible for moving glucose from the blood stream to the cells to be converted into energy.

In type 1 diabetes this does not happen and blood glucose levels rise (hyperglycaemia); this inefficient use of glucose results in a person experiencing increased thirst (glucose leaks into the urine, causing the kidneys to excrete water), weight loss (though appetite often increases as the body tries to metabolise energy from food) and tiredness (CKS, 2014c). Over time even mildly elevated levels of glucose in the blood stream can cause damage to the blood vessels, resulting in atheroma, visual disturbances due to damage to the small vessels of the retina and poor circulation, both peripheral and central.

Further reading

Care Quality Commission (2014) *From the Pond in to the Sea: Children's Transition to Adult Health Services*. Gallowgate: Care Quality Commission.
Key report on the issue of transition.

Drennan, V and Goodman, C (2014) *Oxford Handbook of Primary Care and Community Nursing*, 2nd edn. Oxford: Oxford University Press.
Contains a useful chapter on the care of people with LTCs, including signs and symptoms and management.

Useful websites

www.nice.org.uk/about/what-we-do/evidence-services/clinical-knowledge-summaries
A reliable source of practical evidence-based information on a range of common conditions managed in primary care.

www.cafamily.org.uk
This is a UK-wide charity providing information and support for families who are living with a disabled child.

www.bma.org.uk/qofguidance
This page on the British Medical Association website gives the most up-to-date information and guidance for the Quality Outcome Framework.

Chapter 2
The therapeutic relationship in long term conditions

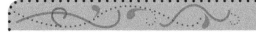

NMC Standards for Pre-registration Nursing Education

This chapter will address the following competencies:

Domain 2: Communication and interpersonal skills
1. All nurses must build partnerships and therapeutic relationships through safe, effective and non-discriminatory communication. They must take account of individual differences, capabilities and needs.
5. All nurses must use therapeutic principles to engage, maintain and, where appropriate, disengage from professional caring relationships with people of all ages, and must always respect professional boundaries.

Domain 4: Leadership, management and team working
4. All nurses must be self-aware and recognise how their own values, principles and assumptions may affect their practice. They must maintain their own personal and professional development, learning from experience, through supervision, feedback, reflection and evaluation.

NMC Essential Skills Clusters

This chapter will address the following ESCs:

Cluster: Care, compassion and communication
1. As partners in the care process, people can trust a newly registered graduate nurse to provide collaborative care based on the highest standards, knowledge and competence.

By the first progression point:
5. Is able to engage with people and build caring professional relationships.

By the second progression point:
6. Forms appropriate and constructive professional relationships with families and other carers.

By entry to the register:
11. Acts as a role model in developing trusting relationships, within professional boundaries.

(Continued)

(Continued)

12. Recognises and acts to overcome barriers in developing effective relationships with service users and carers.

6. People can trust the newly registered graduate nurse to engage therapeutically and actively listen to their needs and concerns, responding using skills that are helpful, providing information that is clear, accurate, meaningful and free from jargon.

By the first progression point:
1. Communicates effectively both orally and in writing, so that the meaning is always clear.

By the second progression point:
6. Uses strategies to enhance communication and remove barriers to effective communication, minimising risk to people from lack of or poor communication.

By entry to the register:
11. Is proactive and creative in enhancing communication and understanding.
12. Uses the skills of active listening and questioning, paraphrasing and reflection to support a therapeutic intervention.

Chapter aims

After reading this chapter you will be able to:

- identify and describe the components of the therapeutic relationship;
- explain the importance of engaging in a therapeutic relationship with people living with LTCs and, if required, their carer and family;
- understand the components of emotional intelligence (EI) and its relevance to the care and management of those living with LTCs;
- recognise the importance of ensuring person-focused communication in the care and management of those living with LTCs.

Introduction

Cure sometimes: treat often: comfort always.

(Hippocrates 460–370 BC)

I will remember that there is art to medicine as well as science, and that warmth, sympathy, and understanding may outweigh the surgeon's knife or the chemist's drug.

(Hippocratic oath – modern version)

Engaging in, developing and maintaining caring and compassionate therapeutic relationships is at the heart of effective nursing care. Doing this allows you to provide person-centred, individualised nursing care. The Nursing and Midwifery Council (NMC) places therapeutic relationships and communication at the heart of nursing practice and this is reflected in the current *Code* (2015).

Those living with one or more LTCs can be in contact with healthcare professionals on many occasions and over a long period of time; this may take the form of a review with their practice nurse or when receiving in-patient care due to an exacerbation. At all stages of a person's journey a key element of their care is your ability to foster holistic person-centred care, promoting **concordance** with treatment and management regimes, foster **autonomy** in managing their own condition and increasing their satisfaction with their care. The development and maintenance of a person-centred therapeutic relationship is central to this: this may involve not only forming a relationship with the individual but also their family and carers. For those living with an LTC, and those caring for them, it may not be the 'what' of the treatment (e.g. the intravenous antibiotics for a chest infection) the person remembers but the 'how' of the treatment. 'How' the treatment was delivered, were they listened to, was the treatment explained to them, was a friendly face there, did they feel understood? To support you in your delivery of 'meaningful' care to those living with an LTC this chapter will assist you in your development of the knowledge and skills required to successfully develop an effective therapeutic relationship with those requiring your care. In order to do this the chapter will help you to develop your knowledge, skills and attributes in relation to understanding what a therapeutic relationship is, emotional intelligence and the relationship you have with carers. Some specific communication strategies useful when caring for those living with an LTC are also addressed.

Case study: Bill

Bill and his wife were struggling to manage his long term conditions (angina and COPD); through working with Bill's community matron they have become more actively involved in the management of Bill's cardiac and lung problems. Both Bill and his wife have regained their confidence and are now able to live more independently. Bill told his story to Patient Voices, a programme founded to support the telling of individuals' stories of health and social care. Figure 2.1 is a word cloud of Bill's story, allowing you to see the words that appeared most frequently.

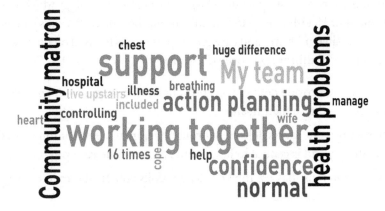

Figure 2.1: Bill's word cloud

(Source: Patient Voices website, reproduced with permission)

*To listen to Bill's story follow the link: **www.patientvoices.org.uk/flv/0029pv384.htm***

An effective therapeutic relationship enables us to *work together* as a *team* with individuals and their carers. This will improve their *confidence* in their ability to *manage* their condition. To *support* this the qualities of care and compassion should be present in everything you do.

Care and compassion

Since the publication of the report into the events at Mid Staffordshire NHS Trust between 2005 and 2008 (2013) the care provided by the NHS has been subject to many reviews. These include:

- The Cavendish Review (2013) *An Independent Review into Healthcare Assistants and Support Workers in the NHS and Social Care Settings.*
- Sir Bruce Keogh Review (2013) *Review into the Quality of Care and Treatment Provided by 14 Hospital Trusts in England.*
- Berwick Review (2013) *A Promise to Learn – A Commitment to Act: Improving the Safety of Patients in England.* National Advisory Group on the Safety of Patients in England.

The main ethos throughout all of these reviews is that care and compassion are human rights and should be enshrined throughout health and social care. People living with LTCs should be equal partners in their care, confident to say when care is not right. Staff should be engaged with the people they are caring for, putting them first and having the courage to speak up on behalf of patients. However it is recognised that this will not be easy; compassionate care takes time and in a climate of pressures on the health system 'time' is a precious commodity. In addition, the use of temporary staff and 12-hour shift patterns can contribute to the 'pressures' felt by front line staff. To address these issues organisations should have strong leadership and governance that values the contribution staff make, and the role of regulatory bodies should be more robust. To ensure that the new workforce reflects these values and is able to meet these challenges, values-based recruitment for nursing and other professions should be a priority.

The findings of these reviews support the *Compassion in Practice* strategy which was published in 2012 (Department of Health and NHS Commissioning Board, 2012). This strategy sets out the 5-year vision for nursing, midwives and care givers, part of this focused on the 6 values and behaviours at the centre of healthcare practice. These are:

- **Care** – the care you provide defines you and your work; it supports the people you work with to improve and maximise their health.
- **Compassion** – how your care is delivered through therapeutic relationships based on empathy, respect and dignity and is central to how people perceive the care you provide.
- **Competence** – you must possess the knowledge, skills and attributes to deliver effective care that is based on evidence and research.
- **Communication** – effective communication is essential to developing caring, compassionate relationships and for effective team work, listening to those in your care is essential to ensure 'No decision about me without me'.

- **Courage** – your ability to speak up and advocate for those in your care, to speak up when you have concerns and to embrace new ways of working.

- **Commitment** – to your patients and communities, your ability to take action to improve the care and services you provide.

These values are of equal importance and underpin the care and services you provide. As you can see all of the 6 Cs can contribute to the development of positive therapeutic relationships.

Activity 2.1   *Reflection*

Take the time to list the 6 Cs and to write down what they mean to you and your practice; how do you incorporate them into your day-to-day clinical practice?

As this activity is based on your own observations there is no outline answer at the end of this chapter.

Activity 2.1 may have highlighted to you the role the 6 Cs play in your communication and the development of the positive relationships you make with those in your care. This type of relationship is called a therapeutic relationship and differs from 'social' relationships.

The therapeutic relationship

The therapeutic relationship is one in which the patient feels comfortable being open and honest with the nurse.

(Dart, 2011, p. 16)

So what is the therapeutic relationship and why is it important to nursing? In 2003 the Royal College of Nursing (RCN) set out a definition of nursing as being:

The use of clinical judgement in the provision of care to enable people to improve, maintain or recover health, to cope with health problems, and to achieve the best possible quality of life, whatever their disease or disability, until death.

(Royal College of Nursing, 2003, p. 3)

Inherent within this definition is the notion of **enabling**. While the above quote emphasises clinical judgement, if you are to truly enable those in your care, and provide person-centred care that meets and addresses their needs, then the development and maintenance of an effective therapeutic relationship is essential. This relationship should be based on trust, self-awareness and empathy; developing this allows you to ensure that the focus of your nursing interventions is on the whole person and their response to the situation (RCN, 2003). Engaging in, through listening and questioning, and developing, through supporting, a therapeutic relationship allows you to recognise the uniqueness of the person (Bach and Grant, 2015). Its success depends on your ability to make and maintain personal/professional relationships with those in your care. The characteristics that define a successful therapeutic relationship (Chilton et al., 2004) include:

- maintaining appropriate boundaries;
- meeting the needs of the person;
- promoting the autonomy of the person;
- ensuring a positive experience for the person.

We will now look in more detail at each of these.

Maintaining appropriate boundaries

Within the therapeutic relationship the maintenance of boundaries is crucial: boundaries define and manage expectation, and they ensure all parties are clear about what can reasonably be expected from each other. The Nursing and Midwifery Council (NMC, 2015) states that you will respect professional boundaries at all times; therefore it is your responsibility to ensure that appropriate professional boundaries are maintained. For nurses involved in the care and management of those with LTCs, the nature of their relationship may vary: specialist nurses may be involved in delivering short term interventions, while community matrons may be involved in longer term care and care planning. These types of interactions will involve different levels of relationship building. Those involved in shorter interventions may focus on the intervention and its success while those involved in longer term care may be more likely to emphasise the development of a connected relationship, where you view the individual as a person first and foremost (Morse, 1991).

The development of a therapeutic relationship is not without its challenges, and for the majority of nurses boundaries are maintained, allowing for the delivery of more person-focused and person-led care. However, given the ongoing nature of the therapeutic relationship in the management of LTCs, there may be the potential for boundaries to 'blur'. Recognising situations when this may happen will assist you in maintaining professional boundaries within the therapeutic relationship; it is about being personable rather than personal, possessing and using effective communication and interpersonal skills while maintaining professional boundaries. Table 2.1 outlines some useful questions (Chilton et al., 2004) to ask yourself to promote appropriate boundaries.

Question	Response
Is the focus of this relationship on the person and their needs?	If the answer is no, use the questions below to ensure that the focus remains on the person and their needs: • Have you undertaken a person-focused assessment? • Were you listening to the person and using this information to plan their care? • Have you let what you believe is right for the person influence their plan of care?

Is this person beginning to rely on me too much?	If the answer is yes, then it may be helpful to consider the following: ask the individual why they are relying on you, discuss this with them and let them know you may not always be available. Relying on one person can promote overdependence, a potential negative where a large focus of care and management in LTCs relates to self-management.
Am I becoming too emotionally involved in this person's care?	If the answer is yes then you need to ask yourself if this is affecting the care you are delivering. (As part of forming therapeutic relationships you invest part of your 'self' in that relationship. Discussing aspects of your personal life may be appropriate if they are used to either help build a relationship or to demonstrate to a person how a situation was managed. However, the focus of that discussion should be the individual and their needs and not be used as an opportunity for you to discuss your needs.)
Is the person and/or their carer/family viewing me as a member of their family?	If the answer is yes, is this appropriate? (Individuals and/or carers may promote a friendship with you as this 'normalises' the relationship and allows them to forget the true nature of their relationship with you. This may be part of their coping mechanism and it may be appropriate for you to discuss this with them in order to find other ways in which they can be supported or accept their current situation. This may be especially true for those who are receiving ongoing care in their own homes.)

Table 2.1: Questions to ask yourself to ensure appropriate boundaries are maintained

Meeting the needs of the person

In a therapeutic relationship the needs of the person are assessed at the outset to identify mutually acceptable goals and who is responsible in the achievement of those goals. The needs of the individual are paramount and should be the focus of the relationship. Actively listening to the person, to find out their concerns, worries, etc., reminds us that the therapeutic relationship is there to benefit the person, not the nurse. Asking a simple question such as 'what is the most important thing I can do for you today?' or 'can you tell me why I have been asked to come to see you today?' demonstrates to the individual that your focus is on them and their needs, rather than your interpretation of what their needs might be. This is especially true when caring for those living with an LTC, where one of the main cornerstones of management is self-care: in order to promote self-care and management you must devise a plan of care that clearly reflects the person's needs as this will increase feelings of empowerment and autonomy.

Promoting the autonomy of the person

Autonomy is the freedom to determine one's own actions and behaviours. A relationship where you encourage active involvement of the individual promotes their autonomy and ensures that they are better able to understand their own situation and take active steps to participate in their care. For those living with an LTC, finding out their level of knowledge and understanding about their condition and how much they want to be involved in managing their own care will allow the level of personal autonomy that reflects their wishes. Many people living with an LTC are experts in their care and will possess a great deal of knowledge regarding their care and management. Indeed, it may be you that is asking the person questions about their care and management rather than them asking you.

It must be recognised though that not all individuals will want to be actively involved in their care to the same degree. An elderly person living with Parkinson's disease may take the attitude that managing their condition is the responsibility of the healthcare team: 'that's what they get paid for', whereas a young person living with asthma may actively seek to be more involved in their care: 'I would like to have access to a nebuliser at home and have a clear protocol written that enables me to manage my condition myself should I have an acute asthma attack'. Neither of these approaches is wrong or right, they are just different. By developing a therapeutic relationship you will begin to know what is right for that person and how to ensure a positive experience for that individual.

Ensuring a positive experience for the person

Meeting the needs of those living with an LTC in a caring and sensitive manner will promote a positive experience for the person. This person-centred approach will not only increase their ability to participate in self-care and management but will also assist them in maintaining a more positive outlook in relation to their condition and future.

In order to promote effective therapeutic relationships with individuals living with an LTC it is important to understand the concept of emotional intelligence. Put simply, emotional intelligence is about understanding your own emotions and those of others around you. Recognising and developing your own emotional intelligence will impact on the way you deliver care; recognising and developing the emotional intelligence of those living with an LTC has the potential to influence how they live with their condition.

The therapeutic relationship and emotional intelligence

Case study: Linda

Linda is 78 years old and has been living with chronic heart failure since the age of 73. Linda started smoking at the age of 19, and has not managed to give up – she smokes 10 cigarettes a day. Since her diagnosis she has made some positive changes in her diet though she realises that she could do more to help improve her health, for example, take some exercise.

To ensure that Linda's care is delivered in a non-judgemental manner you need to have an under-standing about how your emotions might impact on the care delivered:

- *you may feel that Linda is to blame for her current health issues due to her smoking and lack of exercise;*
- *you may feel that Linda is being selfish and lazy and that she should stop smoking and take some exercise to prevent her condition deteriorating further.*

Linda's own emotions may also be impacting on her attitude to her health:

- *she may feel that as her health is already damaged there is no point in stopping smoking;*
- *she may feel embarrassed and reluctant to ask for help in making a change in her lifestyle.*

As you can see from the scenario above there is the potential for our emotions and feelings to impact negatively on our interactions with those in our care. There is also the possibility that a person's emotions can have a negative impact on their condition and how they manage it.

To understand emotional intelligence as a concept we need to go back to Howard Gardner's 'multiple intelligence' theory (Gardner, 1983) to see the first recognition of emotional intelligence, described by Gardener as intrapersonal intelligence. Intrapersonal intelligence is concerned with your capacity to understand yourself, to recognise and appreciate your emotions and to use this information to regulate your life (Gardner, 1999). Acknowledging Gardner's work on intrapersonal intelligence, Salovey and Mayer (1990) developed emotional intelligence as a concept. In their theory intrapersonal intelligence is seen as being part of emotional intelligence. Salovey and Mayer define emotional intelligence as being:

*the ability to monitor one's own and **others'** feelings and emotions, to discriminate among them and to use this information to guide one's thinking and actions.*

(Salovey and Mayer, 1990, p. 189; emphasis added)

Emotional intelligence abilities	Application to practice
Self-awareness	Being aware of your strengths and weaknesses and looking to managing these.
	You may feel uncomfortable when dealing with conflict and recognise that dealing with conflict is not one of your strengths. The important thing is to act on this and to put strategies in place to address this; one might be to attend an assertiveness course.
Self-regulation	Being aware of your 'self' and your emotions and being able to regulate these and not become overwhelmed by them.

(Continued)

Table 2.2   (Continued)

Emotional intelligence abilities	Application to practice
	When faced with conflict your first response might be to become angry yourself: recognising this and regulating your emotions will avoid an escalation of the situation. Working on your communication skills and de-escalation techniques would help manage this.
Motivation	Your ability to use self-awareness and self-regulation of your emotions to inspire yourself and others. Recognising that you find dealing with conflict challenging and having the desire to improve your ability to manage conflict will motivate you to undertake activities that will increase your skills in this area.
Empathy	Your capacity to understand another's situation, to identify with their emotions and to use this to respond in an appropriate manner. By increasing your knowledge and skills in relation to conflict management, and by reflecting on these, you will increase your ability to empathise with and respond appropriately to individuals/relatives/carers that may be angry.
Social skills	Your capability to influence and to maintain and improve interpersonal relationships through the use of effective and supportive communication skills. Through reflecting on your experience of conflict management and through undertaking assertiveness training you have increased your range of communication skills and are able to use these in other situations to support those in your care.

Table 2.2: Emotional intelligence abilities and their relation to nursing practice

As you can see, the difference between intrapersonal intelligence and emotional intelligence is the ability to recognise and respond to *others'* emotions. In 1998 the Consortium for Research on Emotional Intelligence in Organisations (Cherniss, 1998) listed the abilities required for emotional intelligence as: self-awareness, self-regulation, motivation, empathy and social skills (see Table 2.2).

As you can see from Table 2.2, emotional intelligence influences many aspects of nursing care. The utilisation and development of emotional intelligence in relation to you and those in your care will impact on the therapeutic relationship and the delivery of care. Jean (now Baroness) McFarlane, a prominent nurse academic, in 1976 maintained that nursing and caring have similar roots, stating that:

> caring signifies a feeling of concern: of interest . . . with a view to protection. Nursing means . . . to nourish and cherish.

(Smith, 1992, p. 9)

Your ability to form an emotional connection and to hold a person in unconditional positive regard or **prizing** will promote their dignity and uniqueness and will ensure that all your interactions have the individual's best interests at the core (Rogers, 1967), enabling you to provide holistic person-centred care.

Activity 2.2   Reflection

Reviewing Linda's case study mentioned earlier in the chapter how could you demonstrate prizing as it relates to Linda?

A brief outline answer is given at the end of the chapter.

This ability to *prize* within nursing was the focus of Pam Smith in her study: *The Emotional Labour of Nursing: How Nurses Care* (Smith, 1992). Smith found that nurses defined themselves by their ability to care, though in order to protect themselves they must possess the knowledge about how to manage their feelings, a pre-requisite for emotional intelligence which is still relevant to nursing today. This application of emotional intelligence to nursing practice supports the notion of caring that only takes place through the development of a person-centred therapeutic relationship. To support you in the development of your 'emotional intelligence and nursing practice', take the time to undertake Activity 2.3.

Activity 2.3   Critical thinking/reflection

Using your notes from Activity 2.1 and the components of emotional intelligence as listed in Table 2.2, answer the following question:

• *How do the components of emotional intelligence relate to the values of the 6 Cs?*

Using the following questions as prompts, identify your strengths and weaknesses in relation to these areas:

• *If you are feeling overwhelmed by your emotions, what strategies do you use to manage this?*
• *How do you motivate yourself? What strategies do you use to motivate others?*
• *How do you demonstrate empathy?*
• *What communication skills do you use when engaging with people?*

Once you have identified your strengths and weaknesses compile a personal and professional development plan to address these.

To support you in this task there are many online emotional intelligence tests you can undertake, for example: **www.ihhp.com/free-eq-quiz**

A brief outline answer is given at the end of the chapter.

Emotional intelligence and understanding those living with an LTC

While Activity 2.3 relates to the development of your own emotional intelligence, it is also important to be aware of emotional intelligence as it relates to individuals living with an LTC. Being diagnosed with an LTC can result in a variety of emotional responses: anger, confusion and despair as the person adjusts to current and potential losses they are faced with. It is not only the initial diagnosis that has an emotional impact: living with and managing their condition can also have an emotional impact. Reduced coping and increased stress impacts negatively on both a person's ability to engage in the management of their condition and their self-esteem (McKenna, 2007). For example, people with HIV who actively cope with and manage their condition have been shown to experience improved overall health and quality of life (Moskowitz et al., 2009). In addition for people living with chronic kidney disease (CKD), developing appropriate coping strategies has been shown to increase compliance in treatment regimes, and education around accepting and adjusting to the limitations of their condition has been shown to improve their health and quality of life (Poppe et al., 2013). Finally maintaining a positive attitude and displaying emotional responses can influence how effectively people engage in health promotion activities and how well they cope with difficult situations, for example, a deterioration in their condition, and how they manage the resulting stress of this (Telford et al., 2006). To support people to increase their self-awareness you can assist them to identify, express and manage their feelings (McKenna, 2007). This will increase their ability to manage stress and anxiety. Some strategies that you could use are:

- developing their communication skills, e.g. rehearsing important conversations (breaking bad news to their family), and assertiveness skills to ensure that they maximise any consultations they have;
- diary keeping and review, e.g. what was good about today, what was not so good, what made this a good day.

Using these strategies and involving other members of the multidisciplinary team will assist those living with an LTC to emotionally adjust and manage their condition.

The therapeutic relationship and carers

There are approximately 6.5 million carers in the UK involved in the direct care of family, friends and partners (Carers UK, 2014a) and it is estimated that by 2037 this will increase to 9 million. One of the main aims in the care and management of LTCs is to promote self-management and to maintain people in their own homes for as long as possible, supported by primary care services. This increased emphasis on care in primary care, and changes in service provision at local government level, has resulted in many aspects of care now being delivered by informal carers. Therefore carers play a pivotal role in the care and management of those living with an LTC. They are involved in many aspects of care from coordinating medical appointments and managing financial matters to providing personal care and administering medication (Carers UK, 2014a).

This level of ongoing care, day after day, has an impact on many aspects of the carer's life, e.g., financially, socially and health-wise. All carers in the UK have the right to an individual assessment of their needs; this assessment must ensure that their work, lifelong learning and leisure activities are considered. Carer assessments are carried out by the local social services department, though a referral to social services for this may come from another healthcare professional, e.g. district nurse. The assessment provides a baseline assessment of how the carer is coping and what they perceive their needs to be in relation to the following:

1. Any aspect of caring: tasks involved in caring; how is your relationship with the person you are caring for and what practical help do you need?
2. The health and wellbeing of the carer: how is your health, do you have any other pressures, e.g. young children, and do you have any free time?

This assessment needs to be handled sensitively, with the carer being aware that the information supplied will be used to provide support for them and ultimately the person they are caring for. Therefore it may be necessary for information to be shared with other members of the health and social care team. For example if the carer is requesting specific support regarding a nursing intervention then you, along with a community nurse, may provide the relevant support. Other practical support offered may be advising about benefits that may be available, providing information about local support groups, and having access to **respite care** services.

Children who are carers also have the right to an assessment which will focus on: the amount and level of care being delivered by the child and the impact this has on their leisure and school life. It should be recognised that caring as a child can have a significant impact on both the physical and mental health of the child and can impact on their choices and future life achievements. As part of the child assessment it may also be relevant to find out from the parent they are caring for the impact their condition is having, e.g. how does your condition affect your children and how can we support you in your role as a parent?

Despite the fact that this has been the case since the early part of the twenty-first century, evidence shows there is still a lack of available support and information, with 1 in 5 carers saying they receive no practical support (Carers UK, 2014b). A review undertaken in 2008 by Caress et al. noted that few of the studies reviewed addressed carers' needs for information and support, with no studies being identified that focused on strategies to enhance the capacity of carers to deliver effective care. To support carers in their role it is important that you develop a therapeutic relationship to enable you to address their specific needs. These include the need for information and support to undertake nursing-based activities (Bee et al., 2008; Silva et al., 2013), the development of coping strategies and ongoing support that recognise the difficulty of caring for someone living with an LTC (Carmichael and Hulme, 2008) and effective communication and financial support (Silva et al., 2013). The focus of the therapeutic relationship between you and the carer must then address these topics, and any others identified, in relation to the needs of the individual carer and their circumstances.

Coping and support

As a nurse it is your responsibility to have an awareness of the role stress and caring have in the provision of care for those living with an LTC. In your role as a nurse, you can help carers manage stress by increasing your understanding about the situations that can increase carer stress and by providing carers with information about how to manage their stress. Some degree of stress can be productive; indeed stress can increase our motivation to undertake activities, e.g. as a student nurse a stress response to a forthcoming examination may be to plan and undertake a programme of revision. However, it should be noted that too much stress can have a negative impact on our ability to cope. How well the carer is coping with their role should not be ignored – carer stress can have a negative impact on the carer's ability to continue in the caring role (Douglas-Dunbar and Gardiner, 2007). Carer stress is a possibility for any carer; however, those caring for individuals with a mental health condition, e.g. dementia, may be particularly vulnerable. In comparison with the general carer population, those caring for a person with dementia tend to access services less and have higher levels of unmet need (Stirling et al., 2010). In addition they may require specific information and advice to help them understand and manage challenging behaviours (Papastavrou et al., 2007). Stress can affect a carer both psychologically and physically: psychologically it can affect their ability to deliver care sensitively and responsively; physically it can determine their ability to safely provide care, especially that requiring physical interventions, such as bathing.

Carers undertake many nursing-based activities when caring for people living with an LTC and want to be able to carry these out safely and effectively (Bee et al., 2008). Providing carers with adequate education and information regarding nursing activities relevant to them will enhance the care delivered. Some of the key areas identified by Bee et al. (2008) are:

- Medication and pain management – education regarding awareness and understanding of the medication being taken including side-effects, how and when it should be taken, understanding of assessment and management of pain.
- Personal hygiene – education and advice regarding skin observation and assessment and use of pressure-relieving aids, management of continence and bathing and use of technical equipment such as hoists.
- Nutrition – information regarding a healthy diet and specific dietary requirements.
- Management of symptoms – information and advice regarding fatigue, weakness and awareness of a person's mental health status.
- Emergency situations – education and advice regarding recognising the signs of an emergency, e.g. myocardial infarction, and who to contact.

Taking the time to provide practical support and training to carers will increase carer confidence, reduce stress and enhance their coping mechanisms.

Case study: Ali

*Ali is 52 years old, and was diagnosed with chronic kidney disease (CKD) when he was 22. He lives with his wife Nabila; his three adult children all live nearby. Recently Ali was diagnosed with stage 5 CKD, meaning that his kidneys could no longer function by themselves, so he was started on **continuous ambulatory peritoneal dialysis (CAPD)**, which he has at home. As well as working part-time in a pharmacy, Nabila is Ali's main carer. She helps him with his CAPD, medication and managing his CKD. Ali has a reduced appetite, severe itching and he is fatigued. He is worried about what to do if something goes wrong with his CAPD. His current medication is:*

- *Atenelol 100 mg OD*
- *Enalapril 20 mg BD*
- *Nifedipine 30 mg OD*
- *Sevelamer 800 mg TDS (with food)*
- *One alfacalcidol 0.5 mcg OD*

Activity 2.4   *Decision-making*

You are spending the day with the CKD nurse specialist, and are visiting Ali and Nabila (see case study above) to see how things are going. Considering Ali and Nabila's needs and the key areas identified by Bee et al. (2008) what information would you provide?

A brief outline answer is given at the end of the chapter.

As you can see from this case study, Nabila has responsibility for many aspects of Ali's care. This responsibility requires her to have an understanding of Ali's condition, possess good communication skills and have the confidence to ask for support. Additionally, as Nabila works outside the home as well as being a carer, she may be worried about whether she will be able to continue working as her husband's condition deteriorates. It is estimated that there are over 3 million working carers in the UK (Carers UK, 2014b). Since June 2014 all UK employees, apart from those in Northern Ireland, who have worked for the same employer for at least 26 weeks, have the right to request flexible working. Employers must deal with the request in a 'reasonable manner', and assess the advantages and disadvantages of the request. However employers do have the right to refuse if there is a clear business need that prevents flexible working.

Working carers and non-working carers often have concerns about financial security, which can be due to many factors. The extra cost of heating, transport and hospital parking charges and care services can mean that carers, and their families, cut back on essentials (Carers UK, 2014a). Financial support is available in the form of the Carer's Allowance and additional benefits; however this is often a complex area to address. Research by Carmichael and Hulme in 2008 identified the complexities of financial support for carers, especially in relation to the working/benefits paradox, where carers either felt they had to work as benefits were insufficient, or they did not work as this would affect the benefits received. Allowing flexible working to support working carers has the potential to reduce the financial burden placed on carers. Flexible working has been shown to reduce sick leave and improve productivity, benefits for both the employee and employer.

While there are negative aspects to being a carer, for most carers, most of the time, their caring is a positive part of their life. Caring has been associated with positive experiences, for example sharing activities and being together, personal growth and feelings of accomplishment (Brodaty, 2009). Taking the time to positively recognise the role carers play, and the positive and negative aspects, has the potential to increase the carer's feelings of self-worth, giving them the confidence to carry on as their role changes.

The very nature of LTCs make it likely that a carer's role will change over time. Most people do not set out to become carers but rather over a period of time find themselves in that role. It can happen slowly over the course of months or years, due to a gradual deterioration in health, e.g. as a result of heart disease or Parkinson's disease, or it can happen suddenly due to an acute deterioration in health, e.g. as a result of a cerebrovascular accident or other rapidly developing neurological condition. Often the assumption is made that carers are, as they are there and already involved, happy to undertake this role. Developing a therapeutic relationship with carers will enable you to address their changing needs, allowing them to continue in their role as a carer for as long as they wish to do so.

As discussed above, it is important that a person-focused therapeutic relationship is in place if you are to provide effective support to a person living with an LTC and their carer. In order to allow this to happen there has to be an open and honest exchange of information, ideas and wishes. This interactive process echoes that of the therapeutic relationship, and helps to define the need for clear person-centred care and management.

Communication strategies in LTCs

In your role as a nurse caring for people living with an LTC you may be involved in their care at different stages in their journey. This may take the form of helping them to understand their diagnosis, providing them with information during an exacerbation of their condition or caring for them during the end stages of their illness. The questions asked by individuals and the nature of the information given at different stages on a person's journey changes. The aim of this section is to focus on specific aspects of communication that relate to caring for people living with an LTC. To support you in the development of more general knowledge and skills regarding your communication there are many other books available, e.g. *Communication and Interpersonal Skills in Nursing* (Bach and Grant, 2015). When caring for people with an LTC it is important to recognise what some of the barriers to communication may be; see box below.

Barriers to communication

For some of those living with an LTC and for those caring for them there are potential barriers to communication that impact on their ability to communicate and to form an effective therapeutic relationship. This can take the form of sensory impairment, e.g. reduction in hearing and/or vision. Some simple strategies to improve communication in this situation are: ensure hearing aids have batteries and glasses are clean, and to access support and equipment through either Action on Hearing Loss or the Royal National Institute of Blind People (RNIB). For those living with a neurological disorder, e.g. Parkinson's disease or cerebrovascular accident, their ability to use non-verbal means of communication, facial expressions and gestures may be limited. Language difficulties, e.g. where English is not the person's or carer's first language, accessing an interpreter service rather than using a family member to interpret is preferable in this situation, especially where sensitive information may be discussed. As a nurse you may also be your own barrier to communication: in challenging situations we may choose to 'close the patient down', enabling us to retain some sense of control. Changing the topic or engaging in small talk diverts what could be a difficult conversation on to more familiar, easy ground. However, this approach does not allow the person the opportunity to discuss their concerns. Being aware of these barriers, utilising the therapeutic relationship and developing your EI will help you develop effective communication skills.

Due to the ongoing nature of their condition and the focus on promoting self-management it is important that people living with an LTC are enabled to actively take part in the discussions regarding their treatment and management. To facilitate this you can encourage them to use the steps outlined below in the acronym PART; for example, before they attend a consultation with a doctor.

- **P**repare – identify main concerns, prioritise these, and write these down before the consultation. Try to be open in sharing thoughts and feelings, be prepared to concisely describe symptoms, timeframe etc., and bring along a list of any medication.

- **A**sk – ask questions about diagnosis and prognosis, tests, treatments and any follow-up; ensure you get the answers you understand.

- **R**epeat – repeat key points in the consultation, to verify your understanding and ensure consultation has been understood; this also allows the doctor to check your understanding.

- **T**ake action – make sure you understand what is going to happen next, ask for instructions to be written down: if the advice being given is not going to be easy to follow then let the doctor know why to see if an alternative can be given.

Case study: Peter

Peter was diagnosed with Alzheimer's disease about 12 months ago. His main symptoms are difficulty in finding the right words and struggling with remembering directions and the sequencing of events. He has been started on Aricept and has noticed some improvement in his symptoms, though he is very frustrated and has expressed a wish for 'assisted suicide'. He is due to attend an outpatient appointment next week. He wants to manage this on his own, though his wife Sarah is keen to go with him.

Activity 2.5	*Communication*

Read through the case study above. How could you use the acronym PART to support Peter to attend his consultation independently?

A brief outline answer is given at the end of the chapter.

As you can see from Activity 2.5, it is important to listen to the person to understand their perspective and their needs: in understanding their perspective, you will be able to deliver person-centred care. However in Peter's case it can be challenging for Sarah to allow Peter to attend his appointment on his own. Supporting Sarah to accept this and providing ways that Peter can share what has been said with her will demonstrate your ability to develop therapeutic relationships with both of them. Actively listening to the individual is a key aspect of this: Epictetus (Greek philosopher, AD 55–*c*.135) said: *We have two ears and one mouth so that we listen twice as much as we speak.*

Your listening skills can be improved by paying attention to verbal and non-verbal communication, and by asking open-ended questions: these encourage the person to give details and prompt you to follow them up. Use paraphrasing; this involves reflecting back to the person a summary of what they had been saying. Paraphrasing allows you to verify the accuracy of your listening, and accurately demonstrates that you have been listening. Listen first and advise second: if an individual comes to you with a problem you may be tempted to provide a solution; however, allowing the person to talk may allow them to find their own solution. This committed approach to listening enables you to focus on the person, and their needs, demonstrating your commitment to them. An effective strategy that can be used in the care of those living with an LTC is narrative-based care.

Narrative-based care: a communication strategy for LTCs

Story-telling can be viewed as a 'children's activity', yet it is through the use of stories that we understand, experience, communicate and create ourselves. Our stories, like our lives, are constantly changing; they consist of the process of telling the story as well as the end product – the story itself.

The idea of narrative-based medicine contrasts with that of the medical model, where assessment of the person focuses on signs and on gathering a diagnosis. In narrative-based medicine the focus is on the person and uses their narrative to understand the importance of the illness from their perspective: the physical, social and emotional impact of living with an LTC (Charon and Wyer, 2008). Allowing a person the time to present their narrative, by actively listening and using this information as a basis for your care and management, allows for the development of a therapeutic relationship. Some narratives may focus on a specific aspect of a person's care and management, e.g. during a consultation with a GP. Alternatively, the narrative may address many aspects of a person's life, e.g. during an initial meeting with a Macmillan nurse. Asking a simple question such as 'What would you like me to know about you?' at the start of a conversation allows the person time to present their concerns, before you begin to carry out your assessment. Narratives should be written in collaboration with the person telling the story: it may be that you are required to provide some structure to allow this to happen; you can use the following open questions to assist the person you are talking to:

- Can you give me an example of when your problem/concern/symptom affected your life?
- Describe the incident in terms of place, time and others involved.
- Does this problem affect others, and if so, how?
- What were the sequence of events?
- What did this mean to you at the time, and what does it mean to you now?

Allowing the person the time to talk about their situation and recognising the emotional impact that a diagnosis of an LTC has provides the person with ways to manage their situation. This has a positive psychological effect on their ability to manage their condition. The use of the person's story also places the emphasis of the relationship on them and their needs and defines how, why and in what way the person is seeking support.

Activity 2.6   *Reflection*

Elsie is a 77-year-old retired school teacher who is recovering from a cerebrovascular accident (CVA) that has resulted in a right hemiplegia and expressive dysphasia. Working with her speech and language therapist she wrote this narrative while in hospital. How would you have used Elsie's narrative to assist you in planning her care?

No-one really sees me as they walk past. They see the shell of the person I was. This is the first time I have been in hospital and I do not want to be here; if I could talk I would tell them that but I can't. The stroke I had has robbed me of the ability to communicate with the outside world. My stroke has also paralysed my right arm and leg. The doctors do not speak to me but to the nurses – just because I can't speak does not mean that I can't hear. They say I may never walk again – I am not interested in that, I can accept using a wheelchair, after all a wheelchair would allow me more freedom, I could move myself from room to room and decide where I wanted to sit.

(Continued)

(Continued)

I have no-one to come and visit me – you see I never married and my friends, well they are old too and the journey to the hospital is long and tiring. My next of kin is my solicitor. The only visitor I have had is the social worker, Meg. It cannot be easy for her trying to help me when I cannot talk to her; I do try and occasionally I can get a couple of words out, however the harder I concentrate the less I can say. Meg talks to me about going into a nursing home – where I can be looked after. I do not want to be looked after. I want to live independently in my own home. Yet I cannot tell her this, I get frustrated; knock my glass over, start to cry and Meg leaves.

Today the speech therapist came to visit me. Her name is Karen and she took me to a quiet place away from the ward. I spent over an hour with her and she is coming back to see me tomorrow. Karen says it is likely that I will get my speech back, though I will always have some difficulty expressing myself. She says her tests show that I have expressive dysphasia, meaning I understand everything I hear but I am unable to find the right words when I talk. Karen has given me a sheet of exercises to do; she says I am to do them three times a day though I am going to aim for five – on waking, after each meal and before I go to bed. At last a glimmer of hope.

As the answers will be based on your own observations there is no outline answer at the end of this chapter.

As you can see from Activity 2.6 it may not always be possible to obtain a narrative of events from a person in your care, for example those with sensory impairments or dementia. Working with carers and family members to build up a narrative will demonstrate effective use of your emotional intelligence as the use of narrative encourages empathy and promotes understanding of the person and their needs. It may supply us with useful clues that can contribute to a holistic assessment of those in our care, allowing us to set a person-centred agenda.

Chapter summary

This chapter has provided you with an overview of the role of the therapeutic relationship in relation to LTCs; it has also outlined the importance of emotional intelligence as a factor in the therapeutic relationship, both for you and for those in your care. In emphasising how the 6 Cs can be applied to the care and management of people living with LTCs a key message in recent health care delivering is recognised. It has focused on the importance of recognising the role of carers and working with them to support both carers and those living with an LTC. Some specific communication strategies useful in the care and management of LTCs have been discussed and related to clinical practice.

Having read this chapter and worked through the activities you will have developed your knowledge and skills in relation to the therapeutic relationship and long term conditions. You can improve communication with those in your care and their family/carer in many ways. By increasing your level of emotional intelligence you can be yourself, be open and honest, recognise and acknowledge your limitations and take personal responsibility.

By engaging in a therapeutic relationship with individuals and/or their carers you can work as part of a team by listening and responding to their needs. By using communication strategies like narrative-based care you can increase the wellbeing of the person/carer, improve physical and mental state, promote a better adjustment to illness and increase an individual's sense of control.

Activities: brief outline answers

Activity 2.2 Reflection (page 37)

You could demonstrate prizing with Linda through the use of both verbal and non-verbal communication skills, some of which might be:

- verbal: encouraging interaction by asking open questions, using non-judgemental language and
- demonstrating active listening by reflecting back to Linda what she has been saying;
- non-verbal: by making and maintaining eye contact, using open gestures, using gestures that will encourage Linda to talk, e.g. smiling, nodding and by spending time with Linda.

Using these skills would demonstrate you were actively listening to her and valuing and respecting what she was saying. However, to be able to 'prize' Linda fully it may also be necessary for you to recognise and overcome any prejudices you may have regarding how Linda has managed her health in the past. Doing this will ensure that any communication you have is not subconsciously affected by your emotions.

Activity 2.3 Critical thinking/reflection (page 37)

The relationship between emotional intelligence and the 6 Cs:

Emotional intelligence abilities	6 Cs
Self-awareness	Care, compassion and commitment
Self-regulation	Communication, courage and commitment
Motivation	Care, compassion, competence and courage
Empathy	Care, compassion, communication, courage and commitment
Social skills	Competence, communication, courage and commitment

Possible responses to the questions asked:

Questions	Actions	Impact
If you are feeling overwhelmed by your emotions, what strategies do you use to manage this?	Taking time out Talking the situation through with a colleague Writing a reflection on the situation	Improving your ability to manage your emotions Increasing your understanding about your emotions Demonstrating commitment to developing your care and competence

(Continued)

(Continued)

Questions	Actions	Impact
How do you motivate yourself? What strategies do you use to motivate others?	Setting goals and targets Giving myself a reward Being encouraging Being enthusiastic Being honest and realistic	Increased success Increased knowledge and competence Increased motivation and courage
How do you demonstrate empathy?	Making eye contact Taking the time to speak to people Listening and responding Being caring and compassionate Use of touch, where appropriate	Improved therapeutic relationships Increased care, compassion Improved communication skills
What communication skills do you use when engaging with people?	Use of open questions Making and maintaining eye contact Use of non-verbal communication, such as touch Listening and responding	Improved motivation for you and those you care for Enhanced communication skills and therapeutic relationship Demonstrating of care and compassion

Activity 2.4 Decision-making (page 41)

Medication and pain management – ensure that both Ali and Nabila understand what medication he is taking and why, if they do not then explain this to them and provide them with a written summary. Explain that Ali is not prescribed regular analgesia; however should he develop any pain then he can take paracetamol but should avoid ibuprofen. Discuss alternative methods of pain management, e.g. positional changes, hot/cold packs. If Ali does develop any pain explain the importance of assessing the pain; you could encourage Ali to keep a pain diary which can be reviewed by healthcare professionals.

Personal hygiene – explain the importance of keeping the site of the dialysis catheter clean and covered with a dressing. If appropriate, explain the importance of following the instructions provided by the CKD nurse specialist. Demonstrate effective hand hygiene and the importance of general hygiene; discuss the use of emollients to reduce Ali's itching by keeping his skin moist.

Nutrition – discuss with Nabila the importance of a low salt diet and to moderate the amount of protein that is in Ali's diet. People with CKD are not able to excrete urea (by product of protein) effectively and high urea levels can cause itching.

Management of symptoms – skin care and a low protein diet will help improve Ali's itching; discussion about Ali's mood and what to look out for.

Emergency situation – education about the signs of infection, what to look out for and who to contact.

Activity 2.5 Communication (page 44)

To help Peter prepare for his consultation you could assist him to identify his main concerns, to write these down and to identify any specific questions he has that he would like answered. These may relate to his medication and the likely progression of his Alzheimer's disease. You could encourage Peter to share how he is feeling, especially in relation to talking about 'assisted suicide'; it could be that Peter is depressed and would benefit from some treatment, either pharmacological, therapeutic, or both. Help Peter to write down his questions, and remind him to take some paper and a pen, or a dictaphone, with him so he can write down the answers or record them for Sarah. Remind Peter that this is his consultation and that before he leaves he should review with his consultant what has been said.

Further reading

Bach, S and Grant, A (2015) *Communication and Interpersonal Skills in Nursing*, 3rd edn. London: Sage/Learning Matters.
A useful introduction for nursing students to the complexities of communication skills.

Docherty, M and Thompson, H (2014) Enhancing person-centred care through the development of a therapeutic relationship. *British Journal of Community Nursing*, 19 (10): 502–6.
Through the use of a case study this article demonstrates how the therapeutic relationship develops to promote person-centred care.

McKenna, J (2007) Emotional intelligence training in adjustment to physical disability and illness. *International Journal of Therapy and Rehabilitation*, 14 (12): 551–6.
This article discusses emotional intelligence and how it can be used to help people adjust to disability or illness.

Peterkin, A (2012) Practical strategies for practicing narrative-based medicine. *Canadian Family Physician*, 58 (1): 63–4.
This article contains some practice suggestions for encouraging patient narratives.

Useful website

www.carersuk.org
Provides a gateway to all carer UK sites, e.g. Scotland, Northern Ireland and Wales; offers advice and information for carers.

Chapter 3
Health promotion in long term conditions

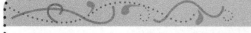

By entry to the register:

8. Is sensitive and empowers people to meet their own needs and make choices and considers the person and their carer(s) and their capability to care.

Cluster: Organisational aspects of care

9. People can trust the newly registered graduate nurse to treat them as partners and work with them to make a holistic and systematic assessment of their needs; to develop a personalised plan that is based on mutual understanding and respect for their individual situation promoting health and wellbeing, minimising risk of harm and promoting their safety at all times.

By the second progression point:

3. Understands the concept of public health and the benefits of healthy lifestyles and the potential risks involved with various lifestyles or behaviours, for example, substance misuse, smoking, obesity.
4. Recognises indicators of unhealthy lifestyles.

By entry to the register:

16. Promotes health and wellbeing, self-care and independence by teaching and empowering people and carers to make choices in coping with the effects of treatment and the ongoing nature and likely consequences of a condition including death and dying.

Chapter aims

After reading this chapter you will be able to:

- explain the importance of health promotion for people living with an LTC;
- understand the influence of health determinants in the care and management of people living with an LTC;
- identify, describe and apply approaches to health promotion in the care and management of LTCs;
- understand and describe the process of motivational interviewing and its role in the care and management of LTCs.

Introduction

Low cost, simple approaches are the key to saving 35 million lives globally (by 2015).

(Dr Robert Beaglehole, Director Chronic Diseases and
Health Promotion, WHO)

While the above quote was written as part of WHO's Millennium Development Goals programme, it is still relevant today. Health promotion is a key strategy for use in the care and management of people living with an LTC. Simple approaches such as reducing the amount of salt in your diet, stopping smoking or taking some exercise can help reduce the burden of LTCs globally. The Ottawa Charter for Health Promotion states that the aim of health promotion is to enable people to increase the level of control they have over their health. Increasing a person's ability to positively affect their health can improve their quality of life by addressing not just physical but mental and social wellbeing (WHO, 2009). In order to successfully engage a person with an LTC in health-promoting behaviour it is important that you know and understand them and their lives. Using the therapeutic relationship (see Chapter 2) as your means of providing person-centred communication and care will contribute to your ability to include health promotion as part of your care and management of people living with an LTC. It should also be recognised that for many carers the act of caring for a person with an LTC can impact negatively on their own health, therefore engaging them in health promotion, if required, will support them in the role as a carer. See Chapter 2 for information on supporting carers and improving their health and wellbeing.

Activity 3.1   *Reflection*

Thinking back to your clinical experience and your role as a health promoter, answer the following questions.

- What health promotion have you been involved in that related to a person living with an LTC?
- How did you carry out your health promotion?
- How did you evaluate the effectiveness of your health promotion?

If you have not been involved in any health promotion intervention then reflect on the health promotion you have seen your mentor involved in.

As this activity is based on your own observations there is no outline answer at the end of this chapter.

Activity 3.1 reminds you about the health promotion interventions you have been involved in with people in your care who are living with an LTC. This might include, for example, the importance of wearing compression stockings and doing daily active limb exercises following hip replacement surgery for a person living with osteoarthritis. These interventions encourage people to learn about their condition, understand the importance of self-care and then to actively participate and be involved in their care. This approach empowers the person, increasing their sense of control over their situation. If we look at the example above it also minimises the risk of post-operative complications, e.g. deep vein thrombosis, therefore reducing the person's length of stay in hospital. In order for your intervention to be a success it is important that you understand about empowerment, health promotion approaches and their use and how to evaluate your intervention. Health promotion should not just be about an individual's health and wellbeing. It should target whole populations and communities. The health promotion intervention mentioned previously may positively impact on the person's health while they are in your care. However, the long term benefits of this health promotion intervention are affected, on discharge home, by the person's family, social support and network and their local environment.

This example not only highlights the integral part that health promotion plays in your day-to-day activity as a nurse but also of the importance aspects such as the environment have on a person's health. This is especially true for people living with an LTC and their carers, where lack of general fitness, mobility or time makes access to services even more difficult. To support you in your ability to promote health in people living with an LTC, this chapter aims to develop your knowledge and understanding of health promotion in relation to the care and management of LTCs. To do this the chapter will focus on developing your knowledge, skills and attributes in relation to health promotion approaches and how to use these to empower people with an LTC to manage their own health condition. Firstly though, to enable you to better support people living with an LTC, this chapter will discuss the factors that contribute to a person's overall health and wellbeing (Naidoo and Wills, 2009) and the influence they have on a person's health, and how **public health** can minimise these.

The influence of health when living with an LTC

As discussed in Chapter 1 the majority of care and management you will be involved in when supporting people living with an LTC takes place in primary care. It may be that, during an acute episode or deterioration in their condition, a person is admitted to secondary care where you are involved in delivering specific care and management. However, on a day-to-day basis people living with an LTC manage their condition either independently or with support from you as part of their primary healthcare team. Their care and management take place in their own home, they live their life in their local community and contribute to the local area. It is important therefore that you have an understanding of how their 'life' (behavioural, social, economic, emotional and spiritual) can influence and affect their LTC and their overall sense of health.

Determinants of health

There are many factors that affect the health of a person and their community. These factors are called determinants of health and can determine how healthy a person is at the present and may be in the future. The health of a person depends on many factors that influence and impact on their life, e.g. genetics, education, environment (WHO, 2010). Table 3.1 discusses the determinants of health (Dahlgren and Whitehead, 2007) and their relevance to your nursing practice.

Determinants of health	Relevance to practice
Age, sex and constitutional factors	These genetic and biological factors are individual to each person; they play a role in that person's health but are largely seen as beyond the remit of public health/health promotion. The Canadian Institute for Advanced Research (2002) estimate that these health determinants influence a person's health by only 15%, with external factors having a much greater impact – 85%. Both national and international statistics on life expectancy demonstrate that, on average, women have a longer life expectancy; however, it can be influenced by the lifestyle choices made by a person and their social and economic status.
Individual lifestyle factors	These can have either a positive or negative impact on a person's health. For example healthy lifestyle choices such as a mother choosing to breastfeed her baby will have a positive effect on her child's health. On the other hand smoking has been shown to be a causative factor in many long term conditions. These risk factors can be seen as being chosen freely by the person; however, a person's social and economic environment also shapes their lifestyle. For example children whose parents, or siblings, smoke are three times more likely to smoke than children in non-smoking households (Royal College of Physicians, 2010). A person's emotional resilience, how they adapt and manage the stresses and challenges in their life, can also influence their health. Adopting positive strategies that develop resilience, talking to someone and seeking professional support early have been shown to improve a person's resilience and their ability to cope with day-to-day challenges (Tebes et al., 2004)
Social and community networks	How well a person can move around their physical environment and feel part of their local community can negatively or positively influence their health and wellbeing. Supportive social relationships, social networks and social participation are known to impact positively on a person's health; however, those who are isolated are known to be at risk of premature death (Dahlgren and Whitehead, 2007). What public services are available and accessible to the local community, e.g. is there a local shop, community centre or what are public transport links like? What support is available from their local community – do they have friends locally?
Living and working conditions	Higher education levels, income and social status are linked to better health, with those in the highest social class (bank managers, doctors, teachers) living on average seven years more than those in the lower social classes (cleaners, train drivers). There are strong correlations between education and health, with lower educational achievement impacting negatively on a person's health. For example, it is likely that people with low educational achievement are in lower paid employment, or are unemployed, and have a lower standard of living. In addition education increases a person's sense of empowerment, their sense of

	how much control they have over their day-to-day life, and prepares children/young people for life. Reducing health inequalities and promoting health for those in the lower social classes are two of the main focuses of public health policy (Marmot Review, 2010).
General socioeconomic, cultural and environmental conditions	These are global and national factors that influence health and are out of control of the person, and in some instances, their country's government. The globalisation of national economies means that countries are influenced much more by what is happening in other countries, e.g., the impact instability in the Eurozone has in the UK.

Table 3.1: Determinants of health (Dahlgren and Whitehead, 1993) and their relevance to your practice

Case study: Linda

Linda is 78 years old, and she lives alone in a one-bedroomed bungalow that she rents from the local council. Her husband died suddenly of a heart attack six years ago at the age of 73; he had gone out to the pub with friends and didn't come home. Linda found out what had happened when the police arrived at her house just after midnight. Linda has one son, aged 53, who visits her twice a week and takes her shopping and to any appointments that she may have.

Linda has a long history of hypertension; it is likely that she developed hypertension during her pregnancy, but this was not diagnosed until Linda was in her 60s when she presented to her GP with occasional chest pain and breathlessness. Linda put this down to anxiety about her job – she was working in the catering department at the local hospital. Following a series of investigations, physical examination, EEG, and BNP (brain natriuretic peptide) blood test Linda was diagnosed with heart failure and was prescribed a diuretic, an ACE inhibitor and a beta blocker.

Linda has been living with heart failure for the past 10 years and has tried to make some changes in her lifestyle; she has changed her diet, but still smokes (10 a day) and is reluctant to take much exercise. She does not like going out on her own as she is anxious that she may become unwell. Linda used to enjoy attending the local lunch club regularly, however she has stopped attending this due to her anxiety about becoming unwell. This has led Linda to become isolated from her local community and she has recently begun to feel that she is a burden on her son.

Activity 3.2   *Critical thinking*

Read Linda's case study above and consider how her current situation might influence, either negatively or positively, the determinants of health listed in Table 3.1.

A brief outline answer is given at the end of the chapter.

As Activity 3.2 demonstrates, determinants of health are personal to individuals and their situation and can have both a negative and positive effect on a person's health. As a result there can be large variations in the health of different groups within the population. For example, in 2010–2012 male life expectancy at birth was highest in East Dorset at 82.9 years and lowest in Glasgow City at 72.6 years (Office of National Statistics (ONS), 2014). If there are no changes to mortality rates from those in 2010–2012, then 91% of boys in East Dorset will reach their 65th birthday, whereas in Glasgow City this percentage is only 75% (ONS, 2014). It is these inequalities in the health of the population, and how to minimise the impact of them, that is the remit of public health.

Public health is proactive rather than reactive. On the whole the NHS provides services that are reactive. This is especially true of secondary care services, in that they respond to a person's health care needs through the services they provide, e.g., surgery for a person with acute appendicitis. Health promotion and health education are seen as part of the service, but the main focus is on responding to a person's healthcare needs. Public health on the other hand is proactive, with its services aimed at early diagnosis, preventative treatment and the development of social policy to ensure all people have a standard of living that supports the maintenance of their health. This might include epidemiology, in relation to an outbreak of ebola or influenza; policy analysis for tobacco misuse; and the influence employment, housing, food and nutrition have on health (Knai, 2009). In all countries in the UK, public health is a high priority on the health agenda with each national government's public health strategy focused on reducing health inequalities. Web links to each country's strategy for reducing health inequalities can be found at the end of this chapter. Having an understanding of the determinants of health and the role public health has in minimising health equalities will enable you to provide effective health promotion for people living with an LTC.

Health promotion and LTCs

> Health promotion is the process of enabling people to increase control over, and to improve, their health. It moves beyond a focus on individual behaviour towards a wide range of social and environmental factors.

(WHO, 2010)

As a nurse caring for people living with an LTC, the health promotion you deliver will focus on improving that person's health whatever the stage of their disease progression. Health promotion will be a part of your care and management from diagnosis through to the palliative stages of their illness. In the early stages of a diagnosis your health promotion may focus on supporting the person to increase their knowledge and understanding about their LTC and how to manage their symptoms so that they can minimise the risk of long term complications. For example educating a person with diabetes how best to maintain optimum blood glucose control (HbA_{1C}) and how this will, in turn, help to reduce the likelihood of them developing diabetic peripheral neuropathy. As a person's LTC progresses the health promotion activities you support the person to engage in may be aimed at restoring their highest level of physical, social and emotional function following an exacerbation. For example for a person living with COPD this may focus on pulmonary rehabilitation and supporting them to engage in some level of physical activity that maintains their lung function. Finally, in the palliative stages of their illness, the health promotion implemented could focus on improving their quality of life, in relation to symptom management through effective use of both pharmacological and non-pharmacological means, e.g., massage, acupuncture. While health promotion may be part of your care and management at different times in a person's health journey, and have a very different focus as a result, the underlying principles remain the same. The process of working together with a person living with an LTC relies on that person being able to understand and to act on the information you provide and use this to maintain and maximise their health. This level of engagement will allow the person to actively participate in the health promotion process, empowering them to take control of their health and wellbeing. The ability of a person to do this is dependent on their level of health literacy, that is, their capability to access, understand and use information to maintain their health (Sykes et al., 2013). Nutbeam (2000, p. 264) describes health literacy as follows:

> *Health literacy is more than being able to read pamphlets and make appointments. By improving people's access to health information and their capacity to use it effectively, health literacy is crucial to empowerment.*

By improving health literacy there is the potential to motivate people and to empower them to take a more active role in managing their health. Low health literacy can have a negative effect on a person's ability to engage in health promotion and ultimately on their health. To address this, in England and Wales, the DH and the Department for Business, Innovation and Skills jointly fund the Skilled for Health Programme (Excellence Gateway, 2015). By embedding language, literacy and numeracy into health improvement topics (e.g. healthy eating), the benefits are two-fold. Participants on the programme gain knowledge and understanding in relation to healthy eating but also improve their level of ability in language, literacy and numeracy. It is important therefore that you present health promotion information in a format and manner that is relevant to the person, their level of health literacy and their situation. A person's level of health literacy will also influence what approach you use to deliver the health promotion intervention.

Approaches to health promotion

As your reflections from Activity 3.1 may suggest, how you use health promotion activities varies; you may use different approaches at different times depending on what the aim of the health promotion is. For example you may use the education model when teaching a person how to administer their medication correctly or you may use the behaviour change model when supporting a person to make a change in their behaviour by reducing the amount of alcohol they drink. Being able to use a variety of approaches is particularly relevant when you are working with people living with an LTC who may require health promotion to be delivered using more than one approach and over a long period of time. In order to provide health promotion to what can be a complex group of people, and in a way that is meaningful, it is important to have an understanding of these approaches and their relevance in the care and management of people living with an LTC. The focus on health promotion here is in relation to the care and management of LTCs. For other aspects of health promotion, see the further reading list at the end of this chapter.

Medical approach

The medical approach is aimed at populations or groups of people and endeavours to prevent ill health and premature death. It can take the form of primary prevention – prevention of the onset of disease, e.g. through vaccination programmes. Secondary prevention addresses disease progression through the use of screening, e.g. cervical screening programmes, and tertiary prevention focuses on reducing further disability in those who are already ill, e.g. cardiac rehabilitation programmes. The aim of these interventions is to minimise the risk of the population developing specific conditions and they are based on the **epidemiology** of these diseases. The success of these interventions is dependent on people accessing vaccination programmes and screening and evaluated through the analysis of data, indicating a reduction in disease rates and associated mortality. The medical approach is clearly focused on minimising the impact of disease, of which there have been some successes, including the eradication of smallpox through vaccination (Naidoo and Wills, 2009). However, living with an LTC is more complex than this might suggest and the medical model does not necessarily address the role that society and the environment play in promoting a person's health. However this approach has a role to play and will impact positively on the health of people living with an LTC; accessing cardiac rehabilitation will maintain and promote a person's health and minimise further complications.

Educational approach

The intention of the educational approach is to provide people with knowledge and information that will enable them to develop the necessary skills to make informed choices about their health behaviours. Unlike the behaviour change approach the educational approach does not set out to effect a change in a particular direction. Rather, it attempts to increase a person's knowledge so that they will be moved towards an informed change in attitude towards their health behaviour. This, in turn, will lead to a positive change in their health behaviour. Educational health promotion programmes are usually led by a teacher or facilitator, and the issues discussed decided by those on the programme. Evaluation of the educational approach may be difficult; people may have increased knowledge and understanding about their health behaviour but may not make the necessary change (Naidoo and Wills, 2009). An example of this type of health promotion approach is the DAFNE (dose adjustment for normal eating) training course for people living with type 1 diabetes. This is a structured teaching programme where those participating in the programme share their experiences and practise the skills of carbohydrate estimation and dose adjustment. Providing people living with an LTC, and their carers, with relevant information regarding their condition and how to manage it can increase their sense of control and empowerment.

Behaviour approach

As discussed earlier (page 54) it is recognised that a person's lifestyle choices can have either a positive or negative effect on their health. The behaviour change approach attempts to encourage people to adopt healthy lifestyles which will then improve their health. This approach believes that people own their health and that people can improve their health by making healthy lifestyle choices; it also assumes that if people do not take responsibility for their own health then they are responsible for the consequences. Making healthy changes, implementing a healthy lifestyle and evaluating the success of this requires long term investment from the person making the change. This means that the impact of the behaviour change may only be noticeable over time (Naidoo and Wills, 2009).

Some people find it difficult to maintain the change in their lifestyle and relapse; this could be due to lack of information or confidence. Recognising this and supporting a person to remain motivated requires the use of approaches such as the transtheoretical model (page 61) and motivational interviewing (page 63) and are seen as integral to any health promotion intervention. Primary prevention has a proven track record in promoting health and wellbeing (Van Gils et al., 2010) with many recent health promotion strategies (such as Change4Life and Making Every Contact Count (MECC)) adopting a behaviour change approach. MECC is a practical strategy that has been developed to support you, and other NHS staff, to use your day-to-day contact with patients and families as an opportunity to promote healthy lifestyle choices. It is through these day-to-day interactions, that promote health and prevent illness, that the vision of transforming the NHS from a reactive 'sickness' service to a proactive 'health' service can be achieved (DH, 2008). For people living with an LTC and their carers, behaviour change approaches can be used successfully once particular needs have been identified and the intervention targeted to meet those specific needs.

Empowerment approach

The aim of the empowerment approach is concerned with enabling people to take more control over their health and health behaviours. This approach will not be new to you. As a nurse you empower those in your care through the development of person-centred care plans. It is a 'bottom-up' approach with the person identifying their own needs and the 'professional', acting as a facilitator, initiating the process and then allowing the person to find their own solutions by increasing their knowledge and skills. Evaluation of this type of intervention is problematic as it is hard to quantify: it is not reflected in the statistics for disease incidence. It is more likely to be evident in the overall affect of a person and their engagement with their situation (Naidoo and Wills, 2009). An example of this might be the use of reminiscence therapy for people living with dementia. The aim of the intervention is to increase the person's sense of who they are and to enable those involved in their care to see more of the person, allowing for planning and delivery of more person-centred care.

Research summary: Reminiscence therapy

Reminiscence therapy (RT) has been used as a therapeutic intervention in the care and management of people with dementia since the 1980s (Cook, 1984). It involves the sharing of memories and uses materials such as old pictures, songs, objects and newspaper articles to trigger these memories. It is suitable for use with people whose dementia is mild to moderate as they are able to access and share distant memories (Brooker and Duce, 2000).

(Continued)

(Continued)

Accessing day hospitals offering care for people with dementia, Brooker and Duce (2000) compared levels of wellbeing in people with mild to moderate dementia. They did this through the use of three activities: RT, group activities (structured craft and games activities) and unstructured time (free time with little involvement of staff). Their results indicated that those participating in RT had a greater level of wellbeing compared with those who had taken part in the group activities and unstructured time. It should also be noted that the group activity had a positive effect on wellbeing though not as much as the RT. Their results suggest that the effectiveness of the RT lies in its ability to enable people with different levels of ability to partici-pate and that using RT prompts a person's full range of senses to be engaged. While this research was published in 2000, more recent research still supports the findings. In Japan (Okumura et al., 2008; Nawate et al., 2008) and Taiwan (Huang et al., 2009) the benefits of RT in people with dementia have been researched. In each study the format of the RT varied: Okumura et al. (2008) focused on themes for each session, e.g. childhood play; Nawate et al. (2008) and Huang et al. (2009) brought together RT and cooking. The results of all three studies demon-strated an increase in participants' cognitive function and overall sense of wellbeing and hap-piness. Huang et al. (2009) showed an improvement in the communication between the care givers and the person with dementia, resulting in increased social interaction.

To enable you to apply the above health promotion approaches to your clinical practice, take the time to read the following case study and undertake Activity 3.3. This will allow you to critically apply the above approaches to a person living with an LTC.

Case study: Sian

Sian Jones is a 20-year-old student who has been living with asthma since the age of 11. After taking a year out after finishing school to work in a local sports centre Sian has just started a Sports Science degree at university and has moved away from home for the first time. Sian enjoys playing hockey and netball and plays for the university teams in both these sports. She is enjoying her studies and is taking full advantage of 'student life'; she lives in a shared house with four other students who are on the same course as her.

This morning during hockey practice Sian became breathless and began wheezing. Sian became concerned as her breathlessness did not resolve as quickly as usual and decided to make an appointment at her GP surgery. You are working with the practice nurse when Sian comes in to see her. During this consultation Sian admits that she has not been taking her beclazone inhaler regularly – she keeps forgetting to do this; therefore she has noticed that she has been taking her ventolin more regularly.

Activity 3.3   *Critical thinking*

Plan a health promotion intervention to support Sian to manage an aspect of her asthma more effectively. Using the sample layout below, complete a chart that includes your approach and intervention and your rationale for your choice.

Approach	Intervention	Rationale
[See activity answers for sample information]		

A brief outline answer is given at the end of the chapter.

In participating in Activity 3.3 it may have been evident that your intervention incorporated more than one health promotion approach. Taking the time to consider your rationale will have supported you to think more critically about your choice, promoting evidence-based practice. In addition it will support the development of your problem-solving skills, allowing you to apply these principles to other clinical situations.

Motivation and health promotion

Dixon (2008) recognises that the success, or not, of a health promotion intervention can relate to how motivated a person is to participate and, in turn, how committed they are to making the change. It can be seen therefore that a person's motivation to participate in health promotion can influence how successful they are going to be in maintaining their health change. Motivation can either be intrinsic or extrinsic. Intrinsic motivation comes from within: I have a desire to change my behaviour, I am self-motivated and I know the change will improve my health. Extrinsic motivation comes from external influences: I have a desire to change my behaviour because if I stop smoking I will save money. To maximise a person's participation in their health promotion it is important to understand what factors influence their motivation to change – are they extrinsic and/or intrinsic (Dixon, 2008). One of the more popular models that addresses motivation in relation to health promotion is the transtheoretical approach (DiClemente, 2007): this identifies stages that a person progresses, and relapses, through while making changes in their health behaviour. People can join at any stage and it is often represented in a cyclical way. Table 3.2 describes the stages of the transtheoretical model and outlines some of the strategies and their aims that may be implemented. To assist you in relating this to your care and management of people living with an LTC the transtheoretical model has been related to Frazer, one of the case studies you are following in this book. See the box for further information.

Case study: Frazer

Frazer is 47 and is living with type 1 diabetes. In the past he has not always managed his diabetes as effectively as he should; this has resulted in diabetic peripheral neuropathy. Frazer has an ulcer on his foot that is not healing; and has had extensive treatment for this to prevent amputation. Five years ago Frazer managed to stop smoking; however he still drinks alcohol on a daily basis. Attempts by his practice nurse to encourage Frazer to reduce his alcohol intake and have three non-drinking days a week have failed; he drinks two pints of beer a day.

What stage is Frazer at?	Your aim is . . .	Your strategy is . . .
Pre-contemplation – here Frazer is not intending to make a change in his health behaviour. He may be unmotivated or resistant to making a change, though he may also be concerned about his health behaviour.	To raise awareness with Frazer of the impact his alcohol intake is having on his diabetes.	To provide Frazer with relevant information in an appropriate format; this may be written, audio or visual. You would then revisit this information with Frazer at follow-up visits.
Contemplation – at this stage Frazer may be stating to you his desire to change his health behaviour by reducing his alcohol intake. Frazer may be weighing up the pros and cons of this.	To allow Frazer to see the benefits of reducing his alcohol intake – both in relation to his diabetes and his general health.	To explore the advantages of reducing his alcohol intake with Frazer. However, you will need to acknowledge with him some of the disadvantages, loss of something he enjoys, challenges and increased stress he may face.
Preparation – here Frazer is stating his intention to change his health behavior by reducing his alcohol intake. Frazer now has to commit to a plan that will enable him to change his health behaviour.	To assist Frazer to manage and overcome any challenges to reducing his alcohol intake.	To form a plan of action with Frazer that will enable him to change his behaviour. This may involve providing him with information in relation to alternatives to drinking alcohol, e.g., low alcohol lager, swapping an alcoholic drink for a non-alcoholic drink and how to manage any withdrawal symptoms. Establishing links with a support group would also be beneficial for Frazer.

Action – at this stage Frazer has made a recent change (within six months) to his health behavior by reducing his alcohol intake. At this stage Frazer's new behaviour is established.	To use an effective therapeutic relationship to support Frazer to adapt and maintain his health behaviour change.	To review Frazer's plan of action with him, to provide positive reinforcement of his success to date. To encourage Frazer to maintain contact with support group for ongoing support to enable him to keep his consumption of alcohol down, or even to stop.
Maintenance – here Frazer has maintained his health behaviour change and has reduced his alcohol consumption and has 3 days a week where he does not drink. He has integrated his change into his lifestyle.	To provide ongoing support to Frazer.	To minimise the risk of Frazer relapsing by evaluating his success so far and to plan coping strategies that would limit the risk of a relapse, e.g. relaxation techniques, creating rewards for the new behaviour.

Table 3.2: DiClemente's transtheoretical model (2007) and its relevance to your practice

It should be recognised that the successful behaviour change is not always maintained and that relapses may occur. To minimise this it is important that you ensure that each stage is addressed comprehensively and that the aim identified is supported with appropriate strategies. This will give the person the best opportunity to succeed; however, should they relapse they will have to revisit the stages, paying particular attention to any that were not fully addressed (DiClemente, 2007).The transtheoretical model provides a useful framework for targeting health promotion interventions depending on how ready, or otherwise, Frazer is to change his behaviour. However, it does not provide you with a specific strategy you could use in your health promotion intervention to enable Frazer to make changes. One such strategy is motivational interviewing.

Motivational interviewing: a behaviour change strategy to promote health in people living with an LTC

Motivational interviewing (MI) is a person-centred strategy that, through the use of effective communication skills, helps people to explore how they feel about changing their health behaviours (Mason, 2008). By enabling a person to explore their feelings in relation to their behaviour change, and giving them the time to work through these, it is likely that their intrinsic motivation to change is going to increase. This is due to the fact that they have reached the decision to change their behaviour themselves and have therefore increased their motivation and **self-efficacy**. Your role in motivational interviewing is to understand why a person might resist change, to actively listen to them and understand their motivations (what are the pros and cons of changing) and in doing so empower them to make their change. The skills you would use and their application to your practice (Carrier, 2009) are outlined in Table 3.3.

MI skill	How you would use it in your practice
Using open questions	Using open questions encourages a person to explore how they feel about a particular behaviour. For example, rather than asking the question 'Do you smoke after each meal?', you could ask 'How do you feel about having a cigarette after each meal?' This not only allows the person to explore their feelings but also helps you to understand the person, their motivation and their feelings better.
Active and reflective listening	By actively listening to a person and reflecting back what they have said you can demonstrate that you have understood what the person has said. For example, hearing the statement 'I would like to take more exercise, I have put on some weight over the past few months', and by reflecting back to the person like this: 'You are able to see the connection between your lack of exercise and your weight', you will encourage the person to explore their feelings further.
Rolling with resistance	There will be times during discussions about behaviour change where a person is resistant to what you are saying. In MI it is important that you 'roll with the resistance' and respond in an understanding way. Resistance can be reduced by reassuring a person that they are under no obligation to change: 'I am here to support you to lose weight, I am not going to force you to change'. Resistance can also be reduced by recognising when a person may not be ready to discuss a situation: 'From what you are saying you don't sound ready to talk about this today, shall we discuss this at another meeting?'

Table 3.3: MI skills and their application to your clinical practice

Using these skills will enable you to find out if a person is ready to make a change in their behaviour. If they are ready to make a change then it is useful to find out what changes they feel able to make as this places control with the person. You can help by breaking a major change down into smaller more achievable steps to maintain the person's **self-efficacy** (Carrier, 2009). The use of MI places the person at the centre of the decisions in relation to changing their behaviour. Through the use of open questions you can encourage them to set the agenda. In sharing information with them, by finding out what they know and then providing relevant information you can encourage them to think about how the information applies to them.

This approach encourages person-centred health promotion that acknowledges the role that the person has to play in maintaining a successful behaviour change.

Health promotion and learning disability (LD)

Increasing life expectancy for people with an LD has increased over the course of the last 70 years (Emerson and Baines, 2010) and it is known that people with an LD experience the same range of health concerns as the general population. Given this increase in life expectancy it is likely therefore to hypothesise that people with an LD will, like the non-LD population, develop LTCs as they grow older. Despite this, people with an LD are likely to receive lower levels of health promotion and often rely on their family or carer to identify and communicate their health needs to healthcare professionals (Felce et al., 2008). The approaches and strategies discussed in this chapter are relevant to the promotion of health in this group of people; however, it is important to realise that access to and ability to engage in health promotion may be limited for some people, on account of their LD. Understanding the barriers (Lindsey, 2002) that might prevent people with an LD accessing health promotion will help you to plan and deliver appropriate interventions.

- Learning and communication difficulties – a person with an LD may not understand or appreciate the significance of a healthy lifestyle or understand the importance of health screening. This can result in the person not participating in the health promotion activity or not mentioning when they feel unwell as they may not realise the significance of the symptoms. By providing information in an appropriate format, e.g. a picture book, providing people with an LD with the opportunity to learn about their health and working with carers you will improve your delivery of health promotion to this client group. An example of this is a health promotion strategy aimed at enabling people with an LD to learn about personal and sexual health (Knight, 2009). Topics include contraception, checking for testicular cancer and sexually transmitted infections.

- Poor carer and professional awareness – carers themselves may not be aware of the importance of a healthy lifestyle, and healthcare professionals may misinterpret changes as being due to the LD rather than another health need. By working with carers to improve their knowledge and understanding and by maintaining your own personal and professional development, you will enhance both the health of the carer and person with an LD.

- Discrimination – there is the potential for carers and professionals to undervalue people with an LD and to neglect their healthcare needs. Understanding your attitudes and beliefs, and that of society's, towards people with an LD will influence the care you deliver.

Most areas of the UK have access to community learning disability teams; these teams are available for you to access and will be able to provide you with specialist information, resources and support. A key role of these teams is to advise and support primary care trusts in delivering annual health checks for people with an LD.

Case study: Daniel

Daniel is 30 years old and is living with Down's syndrome. He lives in supported accommodation with three other people who are also living with learning disabilities. Daniel relies on convenience foods the majority of the time, though his support worker is trying to improve his diet. He does not work and takes limited exercise; as a result he has been putting on weight. Daniel is attending his GP surgery for his annual health check. At this visit it is noted that his weight has increased and his BMI is 28 (it was 24 last year). This is concerning to Daniel's GP as his weight gain will increase his chances of developing type 2 diabetes and heart disease. The GP has asked the practice nurse to work with Daniel to reduce his weight.

Activity 3.4   *Critical thinking*

Go to **www.rcn.org.uk/__data/assets/pdf_file/0004/78691/003024.pdf** where you can find the RCN learning disability guidance. You will find this a helpful resource.

- How could you work with Daniel to improve his health?
- How might you best communicate with him effectively?
- What approaches might you use to help him change his diet? What approaches might you use to encourage him to increase the amount of exercise he takes?

A brief outline answer is given at the end of the chapter.

By supporting Daniel to improve his health you will be able to increase his sense of autonomy and minimise his health complications in the future.

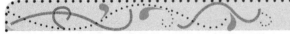

Chapter summary

This chapter has provided you with an overview of the role of health promotion in the care and management of people living with an LTC. The importance of determinants of health and public health in relation to LTCs has been outlined and the necessary role health promotion has in the care and management of people living with an LTC. It has focused on health promotion approaches and how to effect change in a person's health behaviour to enhance their health and wellbeing. Some specific behaviour change strategies that can be used in promoting health for people living with an LTC have been discussed and related to your clinical practice.

Having read through this chapter and worked through the activities you will have succeeded in increasing your knowledge and skills of health promotion in relation to the care and management of people living with an LTC. How you will use your knowledge and skills will depend on where you are working and your roles and responsibilities. Nevertheless, you can increase the appropriateness of your health promotion by using the knowledge and skills developed in this chapter. By increasing your knowledge of health determinants and health promotion approaches you will be able to provide health promotion interventions that address the holistic nature of health. By understanding motivation in relation to health promotion and how to relate this to a person's readiness to change you will provide health promotion information appropriate for that person. In using a strategy like MI you will place the person at the centre of your interactions with them, ensuring that they are driving the health promotion.

Activities: brief outline answers

Activity 3.2 Critical thinking (page 55)

- Age, sex and constitutional factors – It is likely that Linda developed hypertension during pregnancy; therefore there are some biological factors that have influenced her long term health outcomes. While statistically speaking, as a woman, Linda is likely to live longer than her male counterparts, her heart failure is negatively influencing her current health. As her condition progresses her symptoms are likely to worsen, resulting in poorer health and increased contact with health and social care services.
- Individual lifestyle factors – Linda recognises that she does not take much exercise and that she smokes; both of these will have a negative impact on her current and future health and wellbeing. Linda could be lacking in emotional resilience as seen by her anxiety about going out on her own; this could have been influence by the sudden death of her husband and how she found out about this. Working on this with Linda could mean that her health improves as she develops positive coping strategies.
- Social and community networks – Linda does not socialise much; she has recently stopped attending the local lunch club, and this has led to her becoming socially isolated in her local community. However, she does see her son twice a week, so she is maintaining some social links with her family – though she is beginning to feel like a burden, which could negatively impact on her emotional health and wellbeing.
- Living and working conditions – Linda is retired and is likely to be in receipt of both an occupational and state pension; however, during her working life she was employed in a lower paid, lower status job, which means that her overall pension is limited. This could negatively affect her health and wellbeing as she may have to live on a strict budget.
- General socioeconomic, cultural and environmental conditions – Due to global financial difficulties Linda may find that her pension, and any savings she has, have decreased as interest rates remain low.

Activity 3.3 Critical thinking (page 61)

Examples are given here of how all health promotion approaches may be used with Sian.

Approach	Intervention	Rationale
Medical	To discuss with Sian's GP if she should have a regular flu vaccine.	It is recommended that people with asthma, who take regular steroid preventer inhalers, like beclazone, have a yearly flu vaccine administered between early September to early November.
Educational	To provide Sian with comprehensive information regarding her medication – when to take, how to take and why she needs to take it.	Explaining to Sian how her medication works in controlling her asthma, and the need to take this regularly to ensure that the medication is effective, will increase her knowledge about her asthma.

(Continued)

(Continued)

Approach	Intervention	Rationale
Behavioural	Work with Sian to develop a routine so that she remembers to take her medication regularly.	Working with Sian, by asking her to outline her daily routine and encouraging her to identify when the best time to take her beclazone would be, and how she can remember to do this, means that Sian is more likely to adopt a new approach as she has found the solution that fits in with her life.
Empowerment	Provide Sian with education regarding her medication and behavioural change strategies.	Using both the educational and behavioural approach has the potential to empower Sian to self-manage her condition more effectively. Placing Sian at the centre of the plan supports her to take more control over her situation.

It is important that the impact of these strategies are evaluated, therefore it would be important to follow these up in a review meeting with Sian.

Activity 3.4 Critical thinking (page 66)

Both you and the practice nurse will need to consider how you deliver information to Daniel in a format that he will understand. The British Institute of Learning Disabilities provides a range of books focusing on good health which includes titles on healthy eating and exercise. If providing written material, try to ensure that you address Daniel directly, e.g. playing football will help you lose weight and this is good for your heart. Using diagrams and pictures to illustrate the words will help reinforce the message. When discussing either healthy eating or exercise with Daniel speak clearly and allow Daniel time to answer. Provide your information in a positive way, e.g. don't say, 'Don't eat crisps every day', say 'Have crisps on a Monday'. Always make sure that Daniel has understood the conversation; check at the end. Working with Daniel's support worker and the local Community Learning Disability Team will ensure that Daniel is well supported.

Further reading

Bennett, C, Parry, J and Lawrence, Z (2009) Promoting health in primary care. *Nursing Standard,* 23 (47): 48–56.

An overview of the role of health promotion in primary care.

Buettner, LL (2009) Promoting health in early-stage dementia: evaluation of a 12-week course. *Journal of Gerontological Nursing,* 35 (3): 39–49.

A research article exploring the effects of a 12-week health promotion course for older adults with early stage dementia.

Dixon, A (2008) *Motivation and Confidence: What Does It Take to Change Behaviour?* London: King's Fund.

A paper that discusses the role personal motivation and confidence have in relation to behaviour change.

McGrath, A (2010) Annual health checks for people with learning disabilities. *Nursing Standard,* 24 (50): 35–40.

A literature review relating to the use of annual health checks for people with learning disabilities and whether these lead to an improvement in the health of a person living with a learning disability.

Useful websites

www.excellencegateway.org.uk

This is the home page of Skilled for Health, and contains useful resources and information to support you to develop the health literacy of people living with an LTC.

www.gov.uk/government/organisations/public-health-england

This link takes you to an index page where relevant information relating to health inequalities in England is listed; this includes how to reduce health inequalities and makes reference to local initiatives.

www.dhsspsni.gov.uk/making-life-better

This link takes you to the main page where the Northern Ireland government's information in relation to public health and health inequalities is. This includes their main public health framework 'Making Life Better'.

www.healthscotland.com/equalities/health-inequalities/index.aspx

This link takes you to the main page for NHS Health Scotland's information about health inequalities and how the NHS in Scotland is planning to reduce these.

www.wales.nhs.uk/sitesplus/922/page/49811

The home page for inequalities and equalities, this contains information from Public Health Wales Observatory and additional resources relating to health inequalities.

www.makingeverycontactcount.co.uk

This link takes you to the main site for MECC; here you will find resources about MECC, training and elearning activities to support you to deliver MECC as part of your day-to-day interactions with people.

Chapter 4
Self-management and empowerment in long term conditions

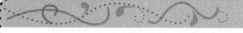

By the second progression point:

5. Contributes to care based on understanding how the different stages of an illness or disability can impact on patients and carers.
11. Where relevant, applies knowledge of age-related and condition-related anatomy, physiology and development when interacting with people.

By entry to the register:

14. Applies research-based evidence to practice.
16. Promotes health and wellbeing, self-care and independence by teaching and empowering people and carers to make choices in coping with the effects of treatment and the ongoing nature and likely consequences of a condition including death and dying.

10. People can trust the newly registered graduate nurse to deliver nursing interventions and evaluate their effectiveness against the agreed assessment and care plan.

By the second progression point:

1. Acts collaboratively with people and their carers, enabling and empowering them to take a shared and active role in the delivery and evaluation of nursing interventions.

By entry to the register:

6. Provides safe and effective care in partnership with people and their carers within the context of people's ages, conditions and developmental stages.

Chapter aims

After reading this chapter you will be able to:

- explain the role of empowerment in enabling self-management for people living with an LTC;
- identify the skills required to self-manage and how to develop these in people living with an LTC;
- understand the role that the Expert Patients Programme has in promoting self-management for people living with an LTC;
- recognise the role that self-management can play in the care of people living with dementia.

Introduction

There is no way you can avoid managing a chronic condition. If you do nothing but suffer, this is a management style. If you only take medication, this is another management style. If you choose to be a positive self-manager and undergo all the best treatments that healthcare professionals have to offer along with being proactive in your day to day management, this will lead you to live a healthy life.

(Lorig et al., 2006, p. 1)

Living with the diagnosis of an LTC can have a profound impact on how people view themselves and their life. Until the time of diagnosis, they may have felt relatively in control of their life and future, but all that changes with their diagnosis. Now they no longer feel they can control their life or future. The aim of self-management in the care and management of LTCs is to empower those living with an LTC, thereby enabling them to maintain as much control over their life and future as they would like to have.

Self-management requires the person living with an LTC to make changes in their behaviour to improve their health and wellbeing. Therefore it is likely that you will use some of the health promotion approaches and some of the behaviour change strategies discussed in Chapter 3 to support people with living with an LTC to self-manage. This is certainly what happened to James, who is living with epilepsy; this is how he describes his experience of living with epilepsy.

> When I was younger my parents were very supportive and tried to involve me in managing my condition, though mum was very protective, however I always felt different – people treating me differently, teachers and so on. When I went to university and I wasn't having any seizures I began to think maybe I can stop my medication. So I did, not only that but I started drinking quite a lot of alcohol; I was OK for a while then I had a seizure at night, thankfully one of my flatmates heard me and came in. That was that, straight off to A and E in an ambulance. I hadn't told anyone at university about my epilepsy, but I could see how frightened my flatmate had been. It was then I realised that I had to take control of my epilepsy, had to acknowledge it, yes it made me different but so what? Over the past few years I have worked hard with a counsellor who specialises in supporting young people with epilepsy. Things are improving, so much so that my counsellor has asked me if I would like to share my story with other young people with epilepsy.

(James, mid-twenties, epilepsy)

In the quote above it is evident that James made a conscious decision to take control of his epilepsy rather than allowing his epilepsy to control him and his life. However, it should be recognised that not all people living with an LTC will feel able to, or want to, participate in their own self-management. For some people self-management of their LTC will not be an option. Bill is 79 and has chronic obstructive pulmonary disease; this is how he describes a visit to the hospital.

> They take your blood, there's no discussion, they're too busy, just a bloke with a machine. Then the nurse tells you there's no change this time, that things haven't altered. I don't want to know more. The GP – we work together – he tells me what to do – but he's the doctor, that's what he gets paid for, and what I paid in for, for all these years.

(Bill, 79, COPD; Corben and Rosen, 2005, p. 3)

While it is evident that Bill does not want to be more involved in his care than he is, other people with LTCs may wish to self-manage their condition but are unable to. This could be for a variety of reasons, e.g. feeling that they are not being listened to, a lack of knowledge and understanding about their condition or their social situation. Engaging people like Bill in the self-management of their LTC requires you to address the underlying reasons for their reluctance to actively participate in their own self-management. By using the knowledge and skills discussed in Chapters 2 and 3 of this book, such as engaging in a therapeutic relationship and using effective communication skills, it will support you in being able to address these underlying reasons for their reluctance.

To support you in effectively accessing self-management strategies for people living with an LTC, including dementia, this chapter will develop your knowledge and skills in relation to self-management in the care and management of people living with an LTC. To do this, the chapter will discuss the importance of empowerment in self-management and how you can, through your actions, help to empower people living with an LTC. There will be a focus on what skills will help a person living with an LTC to become an effective self-manager, and how to develop those skills. The role of the Expert Patients Programme as a means of promoting self-management will be outlined. Finally, the importance of promoting self-management in dementia will be discussed, with some strategies for care being outlined. The terms self-care and self-management can be used to mean the same thing; for consistency the term self-management will be used throughout this chapter.

Empowerment as an ethos of care in LTCs

> *Empowerment is a process through which people gain greater control over decisions and actions affecting their health.*

(WHO, 1998)

Empowerment is not a specific strategy, approach, tool or skill that you can employ in the care and management of people living with an LTC. Rather, it is an **ethos** that will underpin your care and management of people living with an LTC. While you may not be directly involved in many of the self-management strategies available, e.g. Expert Patients Programme (EPP), you can play a significant role in encouraging and enabling people to either learn the skills of self-management or access programmes like the EPP. Empowerment therefore is discussed as an underlying element of your care and management and can be related to all aspects of this. For example, you should recognise that effective health promotion (see Chapter 3) has the potential to empower people living with an LTC to take more responsibility for managing their condition. To appreciate empowerment as part of the care and management of LTCs it is useful to have an awareness of its origins.

As a **philosophy**, empowerment began as a result of 'communities' or groups of people feeling oppressed and powerless. These 'communities' empowered themselves by taking positive action and as a result became powerful and most importantly liberated. Examples of these include the civil rights movement in the USA, rights for disabled people and women's rights; these are examples of empowerment being used as social action. Paulo Freire (1921–97) was a Brazilian theorist who worked with marginalised groups in Brazil promoting literacy. His seminal piece of work, *Pedagogy of the Oppressed* (1970), stated that it would be education that would enable oppressed groups to overcome their situation and regain their humanity (Smith, 1997, 2002). The fundamental principles of Freire's work still apply today and are relevant to empowering people living with an LTC. These principles are as follows.

- Dialogue – engaging in a therapeutic relationship with a person will allow for a framework of mutual respect and collaboration to develop.

- Understanding – using approaches like the transtheoretical model (DiClemente, 2007) and motivational interviewing will ensure that you understand a person's position and their values. Therefore the strategies you put in place will encompass those increasing their likelihood of success.

- Acknowledging those who do not have a voice – having an increased awareness of determinants of health, health inequalities and health literacy will support you in your role as a person's advocate.

- Experience – again through the use of an effective therapeutic relationship, and strategies like narrative-based care, you will be able to listen to and value the experience of the people who are living with an LTC (Smith, 1997, 2002).

The principles of Freire's work have also been used in the field of health literacy (Nutbeam, 2000; Kickbusch, 2001); see also Chapter 3 of this book. Increasing a person's level of health literacy can be seen as a way of empowering them to be able to take control of their condition and play a more active role in managing their condition and their life. The focus of empowerment in this chapter relates to self-empowerment; however, it could be argued that in empowering an individual you are equipping them with the knowledge, skills and motivation to make not only personal changes but also broader community changes.

Activity 4.1   *Reflection*

Empowerment is about supporting a person to become more active and in control of their situation. Reflecting back on your life, personal and professional, think of a situation where you have been disempowered and answer the following questions.

- What was it about this situation that disempowered you?
- How did that make you feel?
- Were there any positive strategies, or was there anyone that helped you to be empowered in this situation?
- How might you use your experience of being disempowered, and some of the positive strategies you used, to assist you to empower people living with an LTC?

As this activity is based on your own observations there is no outline answer at the end of this chapter.

The more traditional relationship in healthcare has focused on the healthcare professional as being in a position of power and the individual receiving the care as being a passive recipient of this care. However, empowering people living with an LTC is about ensuring they have more control over their health and healthcare and that the services/treatment they receive supports them to live the life they want to live (McDonald, 2014). This means equipping them with the knowledge and skills to manage more of their care themselves; this change in emphasis challenges the traditional relationship between healthcare professional and patient as those living with an LTC become partners in their care.

People who are empowered better understand their health condition and its effect on their body and participate more in making decisions about their care. In addition they are more likely to ask questions and to use this information to take responsibility for their health (European Network on Patient Empowerment (ENOPE) 2012) meaning that they only access care when necessary.

You, however, cannot 'give' a person 'empowerment'; they have to want, and be able, to be empowered. A person's culture, age, access to resources, both social and economic, will influence their ability to be empowered (McAllister et al., 2012). Understanding how ready a person is to be empowered and 'active' in their care is important. A Kings Fund Report in 2014 discussed how the Patient Activation Measure (PAM) (Hibbard et al., 2005) could be used to assess how able and willing people are to take on the role of managing their own health. Individuals are asked to state how much they agree or disagree with a range of statements relating to their health, such as:

- Taking an active role in my own healthcare is the most important thing that affects my health.
- I am confident that I can tell whether I need to go to the doctor or whether I can take care of a health problem myself.
- I know how to prevent problems with my health.
- I am confident I can figure out solutions when new problems arise with my health.

As you can see from the sample statements above, PAM focuses on the knowledge, skills and attributes required to successfully self-manage an LTC. As a healthcare professional you have an active role to play in supporting people to develop these and there are certain attributes and actions that can assist you in empowering people in your care (Toofany, 2006) (Table 4.1).

Your attributes	Your actions	Result in . . .
Kindness/cheerfulness	Taking the time to listen	Mutual trust
Experience	Taking the time to talk	Respect
Knowledge	Offering information	Open and genuine
Approachability	Answering questions	Communication

Table 4.1: Your attributes and actions that can result in empowerment

In addition to these personal attributes there are other strategies that can promote empowerment (Toofany, 2006). The strategies listed in Table 4.2 correlate with recent research (McDonald, 2014), which identified that 77% of participants indicated that they should be able to manage more of their healthcare independently at home, but that a lack of support and information prevented this. On a one-to-one level, encouraging people to participate in their care and to acquire decision-making skills, and on a strategic level, implementing more programmes, such as the EPP, and self-help groups, would support people living with an LTC to manage more of their care independently.

Empowerment can be achieved by . . .	
On a one-to-one level	**On a strategic level**
Actively encouraging and supporting individuals to participate	Ensuring that individuals have a say in how healthcare services are delivered
Shifting the balance of power by reducing professional barriers	Promoting joint working and developing partnerships
Helping individuals to acquire decision-making skills	Moving towards a social model of healthcare and nursing
Enhancing communication strategies	Changing leadership culture
Valuing the knowledge of the community	Enhancing communication strategies
Increasing the sense of belonging, self-esteem and self-confidence	Valuing the knowledge of the community
Enhancing skills through education	Expanding programmes such as the EPP
	Setting up self-help groups

Table 4.2: Strategies to promote empowerment in the care and management of LTCs

Activity 4.2 — *Critical thinking*

Revisit Linda's case study in Chapter 3 (page 55). We pick up her story below.

Following two recent episodes of chest pain that both required attendance at the local A&E department Linda's GP has asked for Linda to be reviewed by one of the practice nurses. Using the information you have read in this chapter write down your answers to the following questions:

- How empowered do you think Linda is in relation to managing her heart failure?
- Why do you think this might be?
- How could you assess Linda's willingness to participate more in the self-management of her heart failure?
- What personal attributes and strategies could you use to support Linda to become more empowered?

Once you have completed this activity turn to the outline answer at the end of this chapter and identify any areas requiring further work.

Activity 4.2 will have identified that there are many factors influencing the degree to which Linda is, and can be, empowered – this is true for many patients. The personal attributes you identified, such as taking the time to listen, support the development of a good therapeutic relationship between Linda and you. It is through the use of an effective therapeutic relationship that people living with an LTC can be empowered to take a more active role in self-managing their condition.

Self-management in LTCs

Self-management is the cornerstone of effective LTC care and management; options for self-management should be made available at the time of diagnoses right the way through to palliative and end of life care. Self-management is important both for the person living with an LTC and for the NHS. It is known that people who are not supported to self-manage are disempowered, feel abandoned and may experience increased exacerbations and health crises (McDonald, 2014). It is thought that around 20% of emergency admissions to hospital are potentially preventable, with many of these involving people living with an LTC (Blunt, 2013). Just as with empowerment it is important for you to know where on the self-management continuum a person living with an LTC is. In Linda's case it might relate to information giving to address technical skills, e.g., how to recognise the signs of an angina attack and how frequently she can take her GTN spray. Self-management that includes strategies that address all aspects of self-management (see Figure 4.1) will prove to be most effective as it recognises the multifactorial nature of self-management and that individual empowerment is gained over time and as part of a continual process.

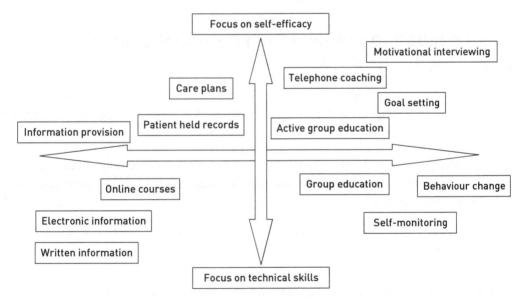

Figure 4.1: The continuum of strategies to support self-management

(Source: de Silva, 2011, reproduced with permission)

Empowerment and self-management will only be successful if you work with people to identify their own needs and support them to make decisions about how they are going to meet them. For any person living with an LTC there are some key skills that are required to support self-management.

Effective skills for people living with an LTC to aid self-management

The skills that those living with an LTC should be developing, to support their self-management, relate to the following subsections (Lorig et al., 2006; Carrier, 2009).

Skills needed to manage their LTC

Any LTC requires the person living with it to learn to do new things. This includes knowledge of the condition and how to manage the symptoms: for example medication management, changes to their diet or coping with side-effects of chemotherapy. Living with an LTC may require more interactions with healthcare services, so it is important that the person knows how to access services.

Skills needed to maintain their normal life

The diagnosis of an LTC does not mean that the person's life has to stop. Managing symptoms, responding to changes and recognising a deterioration in their condition are important factors in maintaining a normal life. It is also important for individuals to have an awareness of how their lifestyle choices can affect their condition.

Skills needed to manage the emotional aspect of living with their LTC

Being diagnosed and living with an LTC can result in a person experiencing emotional changes, some of which can be negative. Learning new skills to develop their emotional intelligence (see Chapter 2) will support them to manage this aspect of their care.

Working with a person living with an LTC to develop these skills will promote self-management, enabling that person to navigate their way through the challenges of living with their LTC (Lorig et al., 2006; Carrier, 2009).

Case study: Joseph

Joseph is 69 years old. He is a retired engineer and lives with his wife Grace who is also retired. They have two grown-up children who live locally with their own families; Joseph and Grace have three grandchildren who they love spending time with. Joseph enjoys going fishing and they both enjoy going walking together; they have always tried to keep themselves fit and healthy. They are both members of their local church and are actively involved in their church community.

Three years ago, at the age of 66, Joseph noticed that he was passing urine more frequently and was having to get up to go several times at night. In addition he was finding it difficult to starting passing urine; initially he put this down to 'aging' and did not seek any advice. Eventually Grace, after many sleepless nights, persuaded him to visit his GP.

*Joseph's GP carried out an examination, sent a blood sample for **PSA testing** (prostate specific antigen) and assessed Joseph's risk factors; being African-Caribbean increased Joseph's risk of developing prostate cancer. Joseph's PSA level was 15 ng/ml; this result combined with his ethnic group prompted his GP to refer him for a transrectal ultrasound guided biopsy. The results of this revealed that Joseph had a **Gleason** score of 7 (indicating that Joseph's cancer is likely to develop at a moderate rate). On discussion with his urologist, two treatment options were mentioned: radical prostatectomy and external beam radiotherapy. Joseph decided to have a prostatectomy and had his operation when he was 66. He has been in remission for the past 18 months; however Joseph has been left with continence problems. He realises he has a lot to be thankful for, but he is frustrated by his situation and he is concerned that his cancer may recur. Both of these factors cause him some anxiety.*

Activity 4.3   *Critical thinking*

Using the information in this chapter about self-management write down your answers to the following questions about Joseph:

- What skills does Joseph need to develop to support him to self-manage his LTC?
- What strategies, on the continuum, would you use to support Joseph to self-manage his LTC?

A brief outline answer is given at the end of the chapter.

It is evident from Activity 4.3 that Joseph requires support from a range of healthcare professionals to enable him to self-manage his condition. Developing Joseph's knowledge and skills will increase his ability to problem-solve and plan a course of action, which in turn will support his ability to self-manage his LTC. Some people living with an LTC might find this quite daunting, so here are some strategies to support you to help people with self-management.

Developing a person's ability to self-manage their LTC

Action planning has been used successfully in the management of asthma and is an integral part of the British Guidelines on the Management of Asthma (SIGN, 2014). Here the focus of action planning in asthma has been on providing a set of instructions for a person living with asthma to use in the management of an acute exacerbation. The key actions of personalised asthma action plans are:

- When to increase treatment.
- How to increase treatment.

- How long to increase treatment for.
- When to seek medical help.

Action points are activated when a certain level of symptom or lung function is reached, e.g. the first action point may be when a person's peak expiratory flow rate is at 70–85% of their best. As an exacerbation of asthma consists of both airflow obstruction and airway inflammation, appropriate treatment may recommend increasing both inhaled corticosteroids and oral corticosteroids. More generally action planning and problem-solving have been identified as examples of strategies that can be used to promote effective self-care in people living with an LTC (Carrier, 2009; Lorig et al., 2014). In this context action plans are set and owned by the person making the plan and relate to specific short term (usually a week) actions.

Let's look again at Frazer, who we met first in Chapter 1.

Case study: Frazer

See Chapter 1, page 7, for further information about Frazer.

Eight months ago negative pressure wound therapy was used as a rescue therapy for Frazer's non-healing ulcer; this was carried out to prevent amputation. Initially there was some improvement in Frazer's foot, however he is experiencing severe pain in his leg and has had further infections, which are now healed. As long as Frazer has ongoing foot problems it would be advisable for him to continue to use an action plan addressing foot hygiene.

Discussing action planning and problem-solving with people living with an LTC involves identifying how these can help them to self-manage, and working with them in the initial stages has the potential to increase their sense of confidence and self-efficacy in relation to self-management of their LTC. The process of action planning and problem-solving begins with the person identifying what they want to accomplish: their goal (Frazer would like to minimise the risk of developing further foot ulcers). The purpose of action planning is to break down that person's goal into smaller tasks (how is Frazer going to achieve this; what does he have to do?). Therefore, while the overall goal might be quite large, the action plan breaks it down into manageable pieces, enabling the person to see that they are working towards their overall goal. Lorig et al. (2014) state it should:

- be reasonable – is this something that the person can expect to achieve in a reasonable time, such as in a week or two;
- be behaviour-specific – giving the person an identified behaviour to address, something they can actually see changing (e.g. rather than saying 'losing weight' say 'no eating after your evening meal');
- answer the following questions: What is the person going to do? How often are they going to do this? When they are going to do this?

- inspire confidence – how confident is the person that they are going to achieve this? They could rate this on a scale of one to ten, one being no confidence and ten being most confident. If a person rates their confidence below seven, they should ask themselves why their confidence is low and review their action plan in a way that will increase their likelihood of success.

When completing an action plan a person may experience problems that affect their ability to achieve what they had set out to do. This could be for a variety of reasons: the overall goal was unrealistic, the action plan was too ambitious or their condition deteriorated. What is important here is that the person does not give up but finds ways to solve the problem that is preventing them in reaching their goal. This could take the form of reviewing their goal or giving themselves longer to complete their action plan. Supporting people living with an LTC to find solutions to their problems will increase their knowledge and understanding of their LTC, increase the skills required to manage their LTC and increase their self-efficacy in managing their LTC.

Action plan		
Goal: to minimise the risk of further deterioration of foot health		
Aim: to monitor my feet for signs of change – every morning this week I will: • *examine my feet assessing colour, swelling, breaks in the skin and pain or numbness;* • *wash and dry my feet carefully;* • *apply moisturiser to my feet.* This week I will avoid: • *walking around barefoot;* • *hot water bottles, hot baths, etc.* This week I will remember to: • *ensure my socks and shoes are well fitting;* • *use my wheelchair when out and about to reduce pressure on my feet.* This week I will be aware of the danger of: • *skin removal, e.g. corns;* • *knocking or banging my feet against objects.*		
What to do if anything changes: • *If I notice any changes in my feet, I am to notify healthcare professionals immediately to ensure appropriate treatment and management.*		
How confident am I that I will achieve this? *8 out of 10*		
Day of the week	*Achieved*	*Any comments*
Monday	Yes	*Inspected my feet today, used a mirror to help me check the soles of my feet, remembered to dry and apply moisturiser after my shower.*
Tuesday	Yes	*As Monday*

(Continued)

Table 4.3   (Continued)

Wednesday	Yes	As Monday, did notice that some of my socks were a bit worn out, buying new ones tomorrow.
Thursday	Yes	Slept in this morning, no shower today but did inspect them, wash, dry and moisturise them tonight.
Friday	Yes	As Monday
Saturday	No	Took Fiona swimming today, had to take my outdoor shoes off in the changing rooms, forgot to dry my feet before I put my shoes on.
Sunday	Yes	Noticed that my there was an area of redness and swelling on my right foot. Contacted the out of hours service and advised to attend, antibiotics prescribed; appointment with practice nurse to be arranged.

Table 4.3: Action plan for Frazer

As you can see Frazer's action plan focuses on practical advice that he can incorporate into his day-to-day activities, encouraging him to adhere to his plan. In addition there are clear instructions for him to follow should there be any deterioration in his foot health.

Case study: Linda (see Chapters 1 and 2 for additional information)

Following her meeting with the practice nurse regarding her recent admissions to A&E, Linda is attending for a follow-up appointment. At this appointment the practice nurse would like to discuss action planning with Linda; during her consultation she asks Linda if there is any area of her self-management that she would like to improve. Linda has said she would like to try to reduce the number of cigarettes she smokes.

Activity 4.4   *Critical thinking*

Using the format of the action plan detailed on page 81, and taking into consideration Linda's concerns, work with Linda to support her to compile an action plan to address her smoking. How would you support Linda to compile an action plan to address this?

A brief outline answer is given at the end of the chapter.

As you can see from Activity 4.4, successful self-management relies on the person who is living with the LTC being able to identify specific goals they would like to achieve and planning and implementing a course of action to enable them to succeed. However, it should be recognised that for some people there may be times where some goals are unachievable. In this situation it is important to support the person to compile another action plan that will enable them to return to their first goal. Alternatively it may be appropriate to find other goals that are more achievable for the individual at that time. This flexible positive approach will focus on what the person can do rather than what they cannot do.

The aim of action planning is to enable the person living with an LTC to successfully self-manage their condition. However, you will have seen that some of the time people living with an LTC will require intervention from other healthcare professionals, e.g. physiotherapist for pulmonary rehabilitation, or podiatrist for foot care. Self-management, therefore, is not about the person living with the LTC managing their care in isolation. It is about the person living with the LTC working with members of the healthcare team, accessing relevant information and education and then using what they have learned to manage their condition in the way that best suits their lifestyle (Lorig et al., 2014).

A strategy to support self-management

So far the focus of this chapter has been on how you, in your role as a nurse, can empower and support people living with an LTC to manage their own condition. However, there are other members of the healthcare team and other organisations who can help promote self-management for people living with an LTC.

The Expert Patients Programme (EPP)

The aim of the EPP is, through self-management, to provide people, living with an LTC, with the knowledge, tools and skills to effectively manage their LTC and maintain control of their condition and life. The concept behind the EPP is that people living with an LTC very often know and understand their condition, on a day-to-day basis, better than the healthcare professionals. Therefore the idea was that a partnership would develop between the person with the LTC and the healthcare professionals. The professionals would be responsible for the diagnosis, monitoring and management of the condition, through tests and treatment. The person living with the LTC would be responsible for adapting their lifestyle, taking prescribed medication and reporting changes to maximise their health and wellbeing (Phillips, 2009). The course tutors are all lay people, living with an LTC, who have completed an EPP themselves and have undergone a four-day tutor training course.

Courses are free and run over six weeks. The tutors do not provide all the answers; instead, the process of the course is to support those participating to identify their own requirements and to look at ways to address them. This is done through the use of goal setting, action planning and problem-solving. The course addresses the following areas (Phillips, 2009):

- dealing with pain and extreme tiredness (fatigue);
- coping with feelings of depression, fear and frustration;
- relaxation techniques and exercise;
- healthy eating;
- communicating with family, friends and professionals;
- planning for the future.

In addition to the EPP there are other self-management courses that either address specific LTCs, e.g., type 1 or type 2 diabetes or mental health or specific demographic groups, e.g., young people or healthcare students. People living with an LTC can either apply to attend an Expert Patients Programme themselves or they can be referred by a member of the healthcare team.

'Living well' for people living with dementia

The *Living Well with Dementia: A National Dementia Strategy* (DH, 2009) emphasises the need for people living with dementia to 'live well'. There are many factors influencing the ability of a person living with dementia to live well and be able to participate in their care decisions. Supporting the person living with dementia to maintain communication channels with healthcare professionals, their family and carers is a key aspect of living well; additionally the use of assistive technology that maintains and promotes independent living is key. As mentioned in Chapter 2 carers play a significant role in the care and management of LTCs; caring for a person with dementia has its own challenges, therefore supporting carers to maintain their role impacts positively on the wellbeing of the person with dementia. The remainder of this chapter will discuss these areas in more detail and their role in 'living well' with dementia.

Communication

People living with dementia should have their hearing and vision checked regularly and professionals should ensure that, when communicating, they take into consideration the individual's ability to communicate. Verbal communication should be person-centred, match the person's level of cognitive ability and focus on the communication ability the person has, rather than focusing on their communication deficit. Listening and adapting your rate of speech, tone and words used to find what gets the best response ensures that communication continues to be a two-way process.

Memory books containing images and simple statements can be used to aid communication and memory recall. A memory book may include a family photograph with the names of the people in the photograph next to them. They can also be used when the same question is asked repeatedly, by providing a simple answer to the question through words and pictures. Another useful resource to use is Talking Mats; this is a relatively low cost communication tool developed by speech and language therapists. They use specifically designed communication symbols that can be used by all ages. People living with dementia have found that the use of Talking Mats help them to remember what they are talking about and remind them of the things they could still do. For carers, Talking Mats helped them to understand what the person with dementia was trying to say by keeping the conversation focused; additionally using them reduced confrontation as the person with dementia could look back at the Talking Mat and see what had been discussed (Murphy and Oliver, 2013).

Working with carers is another approach that can be used to improve communication and support the person living with dementia to 'live well'; this could take the form of carers keeping a diary which could include: changes in memory ability, drastic mood changes, unusual behaviour, health-related changes to sleep, appetite, etc., and any health complaints of the person. These may signify an acute illness, such as an infection, or deterioration in the person's dementia. This information can then be used to review ongoing care plans, address acute episodes and promote person-centred care.

Assistive technology

Assistive technology refers to equipment that may increase the range of activities and the independence and wellbeing of people living with a disability, either physical or cognitive; this includes adaptive aids and environmental modifications (Royal Commission on Long Term Care, 1999). Assistive technology can be used to support a range of LTCs, equipping people with the resources and information they need to self-manage. For a person living with dementia it is important to keep the technology simple and appropriate to a person's level of need. For a person with dementia this might focus on technologies to assist them to move around their own environment. For example a picture of a bed on the bedroom door, a wardrobe with clear doors or a notice saying 'tea and coffee' on a kitchen cupboard can assist a person with dementia to be more independent in their activities of daily living. Using memory aids such as calendars, diaries and a schedule of their daily routine can all contribute to improving a person's independence. Large-faced clocks or clocks that say, 'It's Friday afternoon' rather than the time allow the person to intuitively understand where they are (Gibson et al., 2014). Medication dispensers can be connected to a telecare system that alarms and unlocks automatically when medication is to be taken; they can also alert carers or the telehealth operator when a dose is missed. This technology does rely on the person being able to recognise what the alarm means and take their medication. Therefore ongoing and regular review of the person's ability to use this technology should be carried out.

Telecare is the delivery of care to people living in their own home via computers and telecommunications systems (Gibson et al., 2014). It involves a range of services including household safety, such as carbon monoxide detectors, fire or smoke detectors and flood detectors. Telecare also includes services to ensure personal safety such as fall detectors and bed or chair occupancy sensors. Fall detectors can sense a serious fall and will raise the alarm at the monitoring centre; the monitoring centre will then contact the registered emergency contact number, ensuring that the incident is responded to. Bed or chair occupancy sensors can be used at night; they can be programmed to switch on lights, minimising the risk of falls, an important aspect to consider if the person is known to experience nocturnal wandering. Many of the devices do not require the person with dementia to remember where they are or how to use them. It should be remembered though that devices, such as the fall detector, rely on the person putting them on every day; this may not be suitable for people living on their own. It is clear that assistive technology has a role to play in promoting the independence of people living with dementia; however, it should be used alongside other forms of care such as a day hospital and support groups, and not as a substitute for these.

Mobile technologies, such as MP3 players, can also be used as assistive technology. It is known that, for people living with dementia, music has a positive effect on general function and perhaps most importantly for carers of people with dementia it has been shown to reduce agitation, wandering and irritability (Janata, 2012). Research carried out by Lewis et al. (2015) investigating the impact on carers of MP3 player use by people living with dementia found that the MP3 players were used throughout the day and night with the average length of time that the MP3 player was listened to being 1 hour. During this time carers reported that they were able to catch up on household chores or spend some time relaxing. Participants overwhelmingly commented on the positive effect listening to music had on the person living with dementia, with this having a knock-on effect on their own personal health and wellbeing.

Supporting carers

It is known that people who care for a person living with dementia provide more day-to-day assistance, report increased stress and have less time for family and friends. In addition, those caring for a person with early onset dementia experience increased work-related challenges (Brodaty, 2009). Providing support for carers to allow them to continue in their role is an important part of ensuring a person living with dementia 'lives well'. The strategies discussed above, in relation to communication and assistive technology, can assist the carer to maintain their caring role, providing support and solutions in relation to cognitive decline. Providing carers with training and education about ADLs will enable the carer to provide appropriate physical care for the person living with dementia. Offering carers the opportunity to practise activities such as manual handling and washing and dressing under supervision of experienced healthcare professionals ensures that these activities are carried out correctly (DiZazzo-Miller et al., 2014). This has the potential to reduce the likelihood of injury to the carer in the case of manual handling, and maximise functional independence for the person living with dementia in the case of washing and dressing. Top tips can include (DiZazzo-Miller et al., 2014):

- Nutrition – remember that people with cognitive deterioration do not always recognise when they are hungry or thirsty, therefore always offer food and drink. However keep choices limited so that it is easier for the person to make a decision.

- Manual handling – do not rush, make sure that the person is listening to what is being said and understands what is going to happen. Reduce clutter, make sure that the environment is safe, e.g., no extension cables lying on the floor, and use the equipment that is available.

- Personal hygiene – develop a routine for both morning and evening (this provides familiarity and reduces stress), use the aids available, e.g., perching stool, and if these are not available consider requesting an occupational therapy assessment. If the person does not want a wash, do not argue, leave them, wait a while and then try again later.

Using the above strategies relating to communication, assistive technology and supporting carers has the potential to allow the person living with dementia to stay in their own home for as long as possible and live as independently and as 'well' as possible.

| Activity 4.5 | *Reflection* |

Using a model of reflection, such as the one by Driscoll (1994):

- What – reflect back on a situation when you have cared for a person with dementia and identify aspects of self-management and 'living well'.
- So what – reflect on your feelings at the time and how you feel about the situation now; consider the positives and negatives of the situation and whether any of the strategies discussed in this chapter were used; consider how your experiences compared to those of your colleagues.
- Now what – take the time to think about what you might do differently/the same if faced with the same situation; would you use any of the strategies discussed in this chapter? If so why and how and where could you access further information in the future.

Using a model of reflection will assist you to structure your reflection, ensuring that you stay focused on a specific topic. Using the questions listed will further increase your level of analysis of the situation, developing your ability to critically analyse your practice and the practice of colleagues.

As the answers will be based on your own observations and discussions there is no outline answer at the end of this chapter.

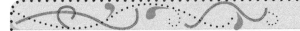

Chapter summary

This chapter has provided you with an overview of the role of self-management in the care and management of people living with an LTC, a key element of recent health policy. It has outlined the importance of empowerment to promote a person's self-efficacy, a crucial aspect of successful self-management. There has been a clear focus on the person with the LTC and supporting them to develop their skills in relation to self-management. Specific ways in which to do this have been discussed and applied to your clinical practice. The importance of self-management in dementia has also been discussed with some specific areas of good practice being identified.

Having read through this chapter and undertaken the activities you will have developed your knowledge and skills about the role of self-management in LTCs and how to empower individuals to take a more active role in managing their LTC. As a nurse, you can improve a person's self-management by developing the skills required to become an effective self-manager. You can utilise goal setting, action planning and problem-solving to enable a person with an LTC to regain control of their condition and their life. By having an increased awareness of some of the strategies available to support self-management you

(Continued)

(Continued) ••

will provide holistic care for those living with an LTC. Self-management is not about the person living with the LTC managing their care in isolation. It is about the person living with the LTC working with members of the healthcare team, accessing relevant information and education and then using that information to manage their condition in the way that best suits their life.

••

Activities: brief outline answers

Activity 4.2 Critical thinking (page 76)

- At the moment Linda is not empowered to self-manage her LTC; she is anxious and concerned that she is becoming a burden. Both of these factors will negatively affect her confidence in her ability to actively participate in managing her own conditions. She is aware that she needs to take more exercise but is worried about going out on her own.
- Linda's late diagnosis may have impacted on her ability to self-manage; she may feel guilty that she did not see her GP earlier; Linda's socioeconomic situation and age may have prevented her from seeking support earlier – she put her symptoms down to stress at work.
- You could undertake the PAM assessment with Linda.
- Being approachable, providing Linda with the time to talk, and answering her questions will increase Linda's knowledge and confidence. Providing information in relation to her heart failure and medication will increase Linda's confidence in her ability to manage an episode of angina herself.

Activity 4.3 Critical thinking (page 79)

Joseph

Skills required to	Strategies to use
Manage his LTC	Providing written/electronic information about continence and what services are available Care plans in relation to managing continence What to look out for that might signal a relapse
Maintain normal life	Encouraging Joseph to self-monitor his condition Group support regarding both continence and survivorship
Manage the emotional aspect of living with his LTC	Motivational interviewing would support Joseph to develop positive coping strategies to reduce his anxiety about his continence and fears about his prostate cancer recurring

Activity 4.4 Critical thinking (page 82)

Linda

It would be important to discuss the aim of the action plan with Linda first; you would encourage her to state her goal and begin to think about how she might meet this. Involving Linda in making these decisions encourages her to actively participate in her care and begin the process of empowerment. A first action plan for Linda, covering week one, might include the following.

> **Action plan**
>
> **Goal: to reduce the number of cigarettes I smoke each day from 10 to 7**
>
> Aim: to identify triggers for when I have a cigarette and to reduce the number of cigarettes I smoke. Each day I will:
>
> - *Remember that my anxiety might increase as I reduce the number of cigarettes I smoke*
> - *Write down information about when I crave a cigarette*
> - *Undertake relaxed breathing when I feel like smoking*
>
> Every day I will keep a smoking diary and will include the following:
>
> - *How intense the craving for a cigarette was, what I was doing, how I was feeling, did I have a cigarette, if so, how I felt after I had smoked, if not, how did I feel after the craving had passed*
>
> When feeling anxious or craving a cigarette I will carry out the following relaxed breathing for 3–5 minutes:
>
> - *Sit in a comfortable chair in a relaxed position with my head and arms supported*
> - *Breathe in deeply, filling my lungs from the bottom as if I am filling a bottle*
> - *Breathe in through my nose and out through my mouth*
> - *Breathe out slowly, counting from 1–5*
> - *Keep doing this until I feel calm, breathing without holding my breath or stopping*
>
> What to do if anything changes: *Contact the practice nurse for further support and advice*
>
> How confident am I that I will achieve this? *7 out of 10.*
>
> | Day of the week | Achieved | Any comments |
> | --- | --- | --- |
> | Monday | | |
> | Tuesday | | |
> | Wednesday | | |
> | Thursday | | |
> | Friday | | |
> | Saturday | | |
> | Sunday | | |

Further reading

Hibbard, J and Gilburt, H (2014) *Supporting People to Manage Their Health: An Introduction to Patient Activation.* London: The King's Fund.

This report discusses patient activation and its role in engaging people living with an LTC in managing their health.

McDonald, C (2014) *Patients in Control: Why People with Long-Term Conditions Must Be Empowered.* London: The Institute for Public Policy Research.

This report outlines the reasons why empowerment of people living with an LTC is a key aspect of their care and management.

Toms, GR, Quinn, C, Anderson, DE and Clare, L (2015) Help yourself: perspectives on self-management from people with dementia and their caregivers. *Qualitative Health Research*, 25 (1): 87–98.

This article discusses the findings of a study exploring the views of people living with dementia, and their family, on self-management.

Useful websites

www.selfmanagementuk.org

The homepage for the EPP and other resources relating to self-management.

www.nhs.uk/IPG/Pages/AboutThisService.aspx

Information prescription service: this is the home page, with external links, that allows you to create information prescriptions about a range of LTCs that include local support and services.

www.nhs.uk/Planners/Yourhealth/Pages/Yourhealth.aspx

The home page for Your Health, Your Way, providing lots of relevant information in relation to courses and support, healthy living, etc., in relation to LTCs.

www.nhs.uk/NHSEngland/AboutNHSservices/doctors/Pages/expert-patients-programme.aspx

Gives information about the Expert Patients Programme (EPP).

www.scie.org.uk/publications/dementia/about.asp

This website focuses on information to support people living with dementia to maintain their independence.

Chapter 5
Quality of life and symptom management in long term conditions

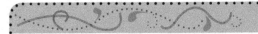

(Continued)

Entry to the register:

12. In partnership with the person, their carers and their families, makes a holistic, person-centred and systematic assessment of physical, emotional, psychological, social, cultural and spiritual needs, including risk, and together, develops a comprehensive personalised plan of nursing care.
14. Applies research-based evidence to practice.
16. Promotes health and wellbeing, self-care and independence by teaching and empowering people and carers to make choices in coping with the effects of treatment and the ongoing nature and likely consequences of a condition including death and dying.

Cluster: Medicines management

35. People can trust the newly registered graduate nurse to work as part of a team to offer holistic care and a range of treatment options of which medicines may form a part.

By the second progression point:

1. Demonstrates awareness of a range of commonly recognised approaches to managing symptoms, for example, relaxation, distraction and lifestyle advice.

Chapter aims

After reading this chapter you will be able to:

- explain what quality of life (QoL) is and how it can be measured and its importance in the care and management of LTCs;
- appreciate the importance of maintaining quality of life of people living with an LTC and where appropriate those caring for them;
- recognise the role that care planning has in effective symptom management.

Introduction

Chronic illnesses come with symptoms. These symptoms are signals from the body that something unusual is happening. They cannot be seen by others, are often difficult to describe to others, and are usually unpredictable.

(Lorig et al., 2006, p. 39)

Many symptoms of LTCs can be managed and minimised by person-centred health promotion and health education and by effective self-management. However, for some people living with an LTC their disease progression is marked out by changing, and often worsening, signs and symptoms. A sign is something that is noticed by other people and is generally objective and can be seen, heard, felt or measured. For example, a daughter may notice her mother becoming increasingly forgetful, and an assessment of this using the Mini Mental State Examination confirms reduced cognitive impairment. A symptom is noticed by the person with the LTC, is generally subjective and cannot always be measured, seen, heard or felt. For example, a person living with eczema may experience a severe itch, though on observation there may be no noticeable cause of the itch. A feature of an LTC may be both a sign and a symptom, e.g., increased pain in a venous leg ulcer is a symptom for the person with the leg ulcer, but is a sign to the nurse that infection is present. The ability of a person living with an LTC to recognise relevant signs and symptoms and to effectively manage these improves their health outcome and quality of life and is one of the key aspects in the promotion of self-management in LTCs.

Activity 5.1 — Evidence-based practice and research

Research the following LTCs: chronic obstructive pulmonary disease (COPD), type 2 diabetes and cardiovascular disease (CVD), and write down your answers to the following questions:

- What are the main signs and symptoms of these LTCs?
- Why do these signs and symptoms occur?
- Briefly describe how these signs and symptoms can be managed.

Some useful resources:

- your preferred applied anatomy and physiology text books;
- **http://cks.nice.org.uk/#?char=A** – this is a useful website for healthcare professionals working in primary care, and provides evidence-based information on managing common conditions seen in primary care.

A brief outline answer is given at the end of the chapter.

As you can see from Activity 5.1, there are many signs and symptoms that require effective management when caring for people living with an LTC. Many people will experience more than one symptom and will be taking medication and using other therapeutic interventions to manage these. Previous chapters in this book have recognised the importance of engaging in a therapeutic relationship, the role of effective health promotion and the importance of self-management in the care and management of LTCs. If someone with COPD smokes, health promotion will play a part in supporting them to change their health behaviour. Working with someone living with type 2 diabetes and helping them to formulate an action plan to change their diet will enable them to self-manage their condition. Through supporting the development of your knowledge, skills and attributes in relation to quality of life and symptom management this chapter will help you to improve the quality of life of people living with an LTC. Using the nursing process and the principles of care planning, pain management and anxiety will be discussed; having an understanding of the principles will enable you to use this process to address other symptoms.

Previous chapters have recognised the role the 6 Cs have in the care and management of people with LTCs. The 6 Cs support engaging in therapeutic relationships and enabling self-management, and remind us that we should be strong advocates for the people in our care.

Quality of life in LTCs

QoL is a term that is used often in healthcare, where the aim of care is to 'improve', 'promote' or 'maintain' a person's QoL. However it is a term that can be difficult to quantify as it can mean different things to different people and can be assessed against many things; for example QoL in relation to health, QoL in relation to employment opportunities. These factors are broad ranging and can be related back to the determinants of health (Chapter 3). The World Health Organization provides a holistic definition of QoL which focuses on how a person sees their place in life in relation to the culture and value system they live in and their goals, expectations, standards and concerns (WHO, 1997). There are many factors that can influence and affect your QoL such as health, both physical and psychological, relationships and opportunities. Over your lifetime it is likely that some of the factors influencing and affecting your QoL will change. It is this subjective aspect of QoL that makes it challenging to measure and quantify. However, it is also likely that there are some key factors that are important to your QoL whatever age and stage of your life.

Measuring quality of life in LTCs

To assist you in your care of people living with an LTC it is helpful to understand how QoL can be measured. There are many QoL assessment scales available: some focus on specific LTCs (e.g. post-myocardial infarction and mental health) and some are generic and can be used across a range of LTCs. Generic scales are useful as they allow you to undertake an initial assessment of a person's QoL, which may or may not result in referrals being made to other members of the healthcare team. One such generic scale is the Quality of Life Profile (QLP) (Raphael et al., 1999). This was developed following an extensive review of available literature on quality of life and by undertaking qualitative research into QoL in people with and without learning or developmental disabilities.

Domain	Sub-domain	Items included in domain and sub-domain	Areas to consider
Being: concerned with who a person is	Physical	• Physical health • Personal hygiene • Nutrition • Exercise • Grooming and clothing • General physical appearance	Peter is currently able to attend to all his physical needs independently; however as his condition deteriorates this may change. When this happens it will be important to maintain Peter's standards.
	Psychological	• Psychological health and adjustment • Cognition • Feelings • Self-esteem and self-control	Peter is angry and frustrated by his current situation and has mentioned 'assisted suicide' to his GP. Peter does not always want to acknowledge that he is unwell.

	Spiritual	• Personal values • Personal standards of conduct • Spiritual beliefs	Peter has mentioned 'assisted suicide' to his GP; he is very family orientated and would like to visit his son in France, but is worried about making the journey.
Belonging: the connections a person has with their environment	Physical	• Home • Workplace/school • Neighbourhood • Community	While Peter is physically independent he relies on Sarah to drive him as he has got lost in the past; both Peter and Sarah do not socialise as much as they used to.
	Social	• Intimate others • Family • Friends	Peter is married and has three children, two of whom still live at home; his family are aware of his diagnosis.
	Community	• Adequate income • Health and social services • Employment • Education programmes • Recreation programmes • Community events and activities	Peter is still working though he has had to reduce his hours, as has Sarah. This has affected their family income but not significantly.
Becoming: achieving goals, hopes and aspirations	Practical	• Domestic activities • Employment • School or volunteer activities • Seeing to health and social needs	Peter is keen to attend his appointments on his own, though Sarah drives him to them. Peter still tries to help out at home by cooking meals, though he does need some prompts.
	Leisure	• Activities that promote relaxation and reduce stress	Peter is still able to carry out the activities that he enjoys.
	Growth	• Activities that promote maintenance or improvement of knowledge and skills • Adapting to change	Peter is trying to maintain his independence and has adapted his working practice to enable him to keep on working.

Table 5.1: Application of Raphael et al.'s (1999) QLP to your clinical practice

The QLP allows for the assessment of the following domains: being, belonging and becoming; these domains are divided into three sub-domains (see Table 5.1). People are asked to rate both their enjoyment and the importance of the items listed in the profile on a five-point scale. With one indicating least and five indicating most, this means that an item can score highly on enjoyment but not on importance and vice versa. Table 5.1 relates the QLP to your practice by relating the profile to Peter (see Chapter 1 for further information).

As you can see from Table 5.1, the QLP recognises the relationship between all aspects of Peter's social, physical and emotional health and how they can affect his QoL. Understanding this will enable you to work with Peter, and his family, to put in place a plan of care that will maintain his QoL as his cognitive function declines. While there may come a time when Peter is not aware of his surroundings and 'who he is', his family will appreciate the steps you take to maintain a sense of who he was.

Research summary: Carer quality of life

With the number of people being diagnosed with dementia expected to increase, and the specific challenges this LTC presents, it is appropriate to understand the impact caring for a person with dementia has. Quantitative research by Rosness et al. (2011) explored the correlation between QoL and depression in carers living with people with early onset dementia (EOD). The researchers used specific QoL and depression scales to identify the relationship between QoL and depression. Their results found that carers of people with Alzheimer's disease (AD) were less depressed than the carers of people with other forms of dementia. This could be due to the fact that those with AD had more insight into their condition and that those with other forms of dementia, especially frontotemporal dementia, display more behavioural disturbances (Rosness et al., 2011) which could negatively affect carer QoL. Having carer responsibilities for children was also associated with depression; this could be due to the fact that people with EOD may have young children with the carer not only caring for them, but also the person with EOD, increasing their caring role. However this was not seen as reducing QoL. Input from community nursing and care teams was seen as having a positive effect on carer QoL; there was someone to talk to and to share responsibility with (Rosness et al., 2011).

Qualitative research by Flynn and Mulcahy (2013), while not explicitly addressing QoL, explored the social, emotional and financial impact of caring for a person with EOD, all factors which are known to influence and affect QoL. The researchers used semi-structured face-to-face interviews with seven family care givers. During the analysis phase of the study, data were shared between members of the team to promote rigour and dependability. From a social perspective it was noted that carers felt isolated, with loneliness being the largest emotional impact felt, due to a reduction in social activities. This was especially evident in younger carers. The financial impact of a diagnosis of EOD was a recurring theme and seen as particularly challenging, as the financial impact had both short (reduced income) and long (loss of pension) term implications (Flynn and Mulcahy, 2013). Finally their research identified that there was a lack of specific services for people with EOD, with the main support available being aimed at older people with dementia.

| Activity 5.2 | Decision-making |

Review the case study about Joseph in Chapter 4, pages 78–9. Then, using the information above on QoL and the questions below, complete a sample QLP for Joseph (using Table 5.1 for guidance). Using the information on QoL and Table 5.1, relate the QLP to the above scenario and answer the following questions. You can either write down your answers or discuss these with colleagues.

- What is affecting Josephs's QoL?
- What areas of his life are being affected?

A brief outline answer is given at the end of the chapter.

As you will see from Activity 5.2, Joseph's diagnosis has had a negative impact on many of the areas that influence his QoL. However, there are some areas that will impact positively, such as his support from his family and his connection with his church. In Joseph's situation you could use your assessment of his QoL to address some of the priorities of his care; for example, practical support regarding aids to manage his continence problems. You can use your assessment of a person's QoL to provide a plan of care that will effectively manage their symptoms and increase QoL.

The aim of effective symptom management is to provide a plan of care to reduce the symptoms a person is experiencing, which would result in an increase in the person's QoL.

Symptom management in LTCs

Activity 5.1 (page 93) has shown you that people living with an LTC will experience many symptoms depending on the LTC they are living with. Effective symptom management requires an appropriate person-centred plan of care to be in place that addresses these symptoms. There are many ways that you can put together a plan of care for a person, e.g. an action plan. Traditional care plans may be either pre-printed or handwritten, core or individualised and may include care pathways. Working in collaboration with the person allows a personalised care plan to be drawn up. This has the benefit of ensuring that the care and management planned clearly meets their individual needs. Rather than achieving a 'best fit' for the person and their needs you achieve a 'perfect fit'. As they are time-consuming to write, however, a compromise may be to use core care plans that are personalised to the individual person and their needs (Barrett et al., 2009).

Medicines optimisation

Having an awareness of medicines optimisation is important as medication is the most common therapeutic intervention used in the management of LTCs. It is known that between 30–50% of people living with an LTC do not take their medication as prescribed (NICE, 2009). This has the potential to impact negatively on their health, quality of life and life expectancy and can also increase healthcare costs. Medicines optimisation aims to change this and is about shared decision-making, promoting a person-centred approach to ensure that people living with an LTC have the best possible outcomes from their medication (NICE, 2015). As mentioned in Chapter 1, many people living with LTCs live with one or more, e.g., diabetes and coronary heart disease. This multimorbidity means that people have multiple medications for different LTCs, and this is called **polypharmacy**. Polypharmacy can be both appropriate and problematic; appropriate polypharmacy is when the patient's experience is understood and that medicine use is as safe as possible, taking into consideration best evidence (Kaufman, 2014). However, problematic polypharmacy is when medications are prescribed inappropriately increasing the likelihood of drug interactions, reducing adherence to the prescribed regimen, both of which can affect a person's QoL (Duerden et al., 2013).

To support medicines optimisation it is important that you understand how people living with LTCs view their medication and what might result in non-adherence to their medication regime. For young people living with an LTC, it might be that they are in denial about their diagnosis or that they feel stigmatised. People who have been on a medication for a long time, and who are now asymptomatic, may decide that their medication is now unnecessary and stop taking it. Older people, or those with an LTC that affects manual dexterity, may find that they are not able to open the packaging. People with cognitive decline may forget to take their medication.

There are many aspects of medicines optimisation, and having an awareness of these will support you in your care and management of people with LTCs. These include (NICE, 2015):

- Medicines reconciliation – the aim of medicines reconciliation is to ensure that the medication a person is prescribed on admission/transfer or discharge from one care setting to another is the same as those they were taking before admission/transfer/discharge. This should be carried out by clinical staff and should involve the patient and their family/carer. A definitive list is drawn up that includes over-the-counter medication and alternatives, e.g., herbal and supplements. Any discrepancies should be noted and this information shared with either primary or secondary care services.

- Medication review – this can take place in any care setting and is usually carried out by a pharmacist. The aim is to examine a person's medication to optimise the efficacy of their medication, to reduce the number of adverse interactions and minimise waste. All medication, including over-the-counter medication, should be reviewed. How effective they are, how appropriate they are and if the person has had, or is at risk of, any adverse reactions should be included. Taking into consideration the person's, and their family/carer's views, understanding and questions will promote a person-centred approach and will encourage the person to think about the importance of their medication and its benefits to them.

Medication reconciliation can promote appropriate polypharmacy and reduce the likelihood of a person taking incorrect medication. Medication reviews can offer people the opportunity to take a more active role in decision-making and the management of their LTC by increasing their knowledge and understanding about their medication.

With a focus on pain management and anxiety and through the use of case scenarios and the nursing process the following section will develop your knowledge and skills in relation to symptom management in LTCs.

Care planning and symptom management in LTCs

As a nurse involved in the care and management of people living with an LTC, using a scheme of care planning known as the nursing process (Yura and Walsh, 1973) enables you to work with the person, their family and carers, to successfully manage their symptoms. Whether you use Roper, Logan and Tierney's activities of daily living model (Roper et al., 2000), Orem's self-care model (1980) or the tidal model (Barker, 2001), the nursing process is the means by which you implement your model. Over the years this process has been adapted and refined: Barrett et al. (2009) have included a further two steps to the nursing process to aid problem-solving:

- assess;
- systematic nursing diagnosis;
- plan;
- implement;
- recheck;
- evaluate.

This six-step process can be remembered by the acronym ASPIRE. When using the nursing process it is important to remember that all steps are interrelated. A plan cannot be made unless an assessment has taken place and a systematic nursing diagnosis has been made; care cannot be evaluated unless a plan has been implemented and rechecked. For the nursing process to be used effectively you must possess effective communication skills, have developed a positive therapeutic relationship, have a sound knowledge of the LTC the person is living with and how the symptoms of this can be managed. Used efficiently and in partnership with the person living with an LTC, good care planning can ensure holistic symptom management.

The management of pain in LTCs

Activity 5.3   *Critical thinking*

Pain is *an unpleasant sensory and emotional experience associated with actual or potential tissue damage.*

(International Association for the Study of Pain, 1986)

(Continued)

(Continued)

> The perception of pain evolved in humans to warn us of danger so we can take action to avoid damage. For example, we withdraw our hand from a flame to avoid getting burnt. However, for people with an LTC it is not possible to withdraw from the pain as the pain may be caused by the condition. To help you to provide effective pain management to people with LTCs it is important to have an understanding of the mechanisms of how we feel pain and the different types of pain. To support you to do this answer the following questions:
>
> - How do we feel pain?
> - What is the difference between nociceptive and neuropathic pain?
> - What are the body's natural analgesics?
>
> *A brief outline answer is given at the end of the chapter.*

As you can see from Activity 5.3, there are differences in the way pain is experienced, whether it is acute and chronic, and in how the pain is transmitted via the nervous system. It is therefore important to know if the person is experiencing acute or chronic pain and whether it is nociceptive or neuropathic, as this will influence how you manage their pain. However, it should be noted that pain is not purely a series of physiological processes.

Pain is what the patient says it is.

(Thomas, 2003, p. 124)

Pain is experienced by people and families – not nerve endings.

(Dame Cicely Saunders)

Pain is a common symptom for people living with an LTC and for many people it is their major concern and for many their pain will be chronic. The Chronic Pain Policy Coalition aims to develop an improved strategy to prevent, treat and manage chronic pain. They recognise chronic pain as an LTC and that the care and management of chronic pain could be improved. A report published in 2011 identified that:

- clear standards should be agreed for the identification, assessment and initial management of chronic pain;
- a campaign should be organised to increase understanding in health and social care professionals about the impact of chronic pain and how to prevent and treat it;
- nationally agreed commissioning guidance should be developed that describes best care;
- an epidemiology of chronic pain working group should be set up to gather data and monitor chronic pain.

Pain has many causes and means different things to different people: it changes during the course of an LTC and its treatment and management vary from person to person (Endacott et al., 2009). This highlights the individual nature of pain. In the 1960s, as a result of her research with terminally ill people, Dame Cicely Saunders developed the concept of 'total pain'. 'Total pain' incorporates the physical, social, spiritual and psychological aspects of a person; these aspects then interact to produce a person's individual pain experience (Clark, 2002). Table 5.2 outlines some of the factors that can influence a person's 'total pain' as applied to Frazer (see Activity 5.4).

Aspects	Influencing factors	Application to practice
Physical	The condition The person's functional capacity Side-effects of treatment Disfigurement	Frazer's foot problems cause him pain and discomfort; pain has reduced his ability to mobilise – he uses both crutches and a wheelchair.
Social	Family issues Loss of role at work Loss of role at home Finances Change in appearance due to condition Sense of helplessness	Frazer has had to reduce his working hours to part-time; this may mean he feels he is not fulfilling his role as 'bread winner'. When out in his crutches/wheelchair, he may have to rely on other people to help him, e.g. by opening doors.
Spiritual	Purpose Religion Meaning Uncertainty about future Hope Fear of pain/death	Frazer is facing the possibility of amputation. While this might address some of his pain, it will further reduce his independence.
Psychological	Anger Delays in diagnosis Coping ability Control and sense of usefulness Failure of treatment	Due to the fact that Frazer has not always managed his diabetes effectively, he may feel that in some way he is to blame for his current situation.

Table 5.2: 'Total pain': aspects, influencing factors and application to practice

This personal construct of pain means that pain is subjective, making an unbiased objective assessment of it complex and challenging. You must remain objective at all times and recognise how your perceptions and the individuality of the person can impact on pain perception. If you use the nursing process to structure your care and management of a person's pain, then undertaking a comprehensive assessment of a person and their pain is the first step to successful management.

Assessing pain in long term conditions

> ### Case study: Angela
>
> *Angela was diagnosed with relapsing remitting multiple sclerosis 11 years ago. She is married to James and has two sons, Charlie (11 years) and Jack (9 years). Over the past 11 years Angela has experienced several relapses of her MS, with two affecting her right leg. Angela's last relapse eight weeks ago has left her with residual spasms in her leg, causing musculoskeletal pain and discomfort. Angela now works part-time as a teaching assistant; James works full-time as a software engineer; recent promotion has meant his is away from home more than previously.*
>
> *Since her last remission 8 weeks ago, Angela is still off work. You are spending time with the MS clinical nurse specialist (CNS) who is visiting Angela. During this consultation Angela mentions her residual spasms and musculoskeletal pain. Angela's pain is due to muscle spasm, caused by increased muscle tone due to nerve damage. This causes the stretch muscles in her lower leg to become hyperactive. Her spasms and associated musculoskeletal pain are worse at night.*

Activity 5.4   *Evidence-based practice and research*

> Reflecting back on the concept of 'total pain', what could be contributing to Angela's pain in the case study above?
>
> What methods could you and the CNS use to assess Angela's 'total pain'?
>
> *A brief outline answer is given at the end of the chapter.*

Activity 5.4 has demonstrated that there are many ways in which a person's pain can be assessed. It may be that you may have to try more than one method of assessment until you find one that is suitable. Consistency of pain assessment is important to enable a clear picture of a person's pain to be obtained. Therefore it is important that the same method of pain assessment is used each time a person's pain is assessed. In Angela's case you could ask her to keep a pain diary. Including Angela's own assessment of her pain alongside your assessment will enhance the overall picture you obtain. For some people, e.g., those with cognitive impairment or a learning disability, ensuring effective pain assessment can be challenging and may result in pain being undiagnosed or undertreated.

Pain assessment in cognitive impairment

Undiagnosed or undertreated pain in people with cognitive impairment may be due to a variety of reasons. In Alzheimer's disease, for example, many of the areas of the brain that are affected, the hippocampus and the prefrontal cortex, are also involved in processing pain (Porth and

Matfin, 2010). People with cognitive impairment may underreport their pain; they may not understand the questions being asked; in addition due to lack, or loss, of communication skills, their ability to verbalise that they are in pain may be reduced (Achterberg et al., 2013). However, people with cognitive impairment can experience the same physical health conditions as those without cognitive impairment (e.g., diabetes, COPD, musculoskeletal problems), and therefore it is likely that they experience similar amounts of pain as people without cognitive impairment.

Many pain assessment tools require the person to verbalise their pain, which people with a cognitive impairment find difficult. Therefore as well as using picture scale tools, using specific pain assessment tools for people with cognitive impairment is important.

- Abbey pain scale – this is an assessment tool for use with people who have dementia and are not able to verbalise. Assessment is undertaken by observing the person and reporting on a variety of indicators. These include behaviour changes, e.g., increasing confusion, facial expressions, e.g., looking frightened and physical changes, e.g., contractures.
- Pain assessment in advanced dementia (PAINAD) – an observational tool that looks at the person's breathing, vocalising, facial expression, body language and how consolable they are.
- The disability distress assessment tool – this is used to help identify distress cues in people with cognitive impairment or limited communication. It describes the person's normal behaviour; for example, what vocal sounds they make when they are content and what sounds they make when they are distressed. A note is then made of what situations are known to cause the person distress. Once completed, this assessment tool can be used to identify times when a person is distressed. While this tool identifies distress it can be a useful indicator of pain.

Working with the person's carer, especially to find out what the person's normal behaviour is, will enhance any pain assessment carried out. This section reiterates that it is the process of assessment and the knowledge and skills you use and not just the assessment tool being used that is important (Endacott et al., 2009).

Having used a holistic approach to assessing Angela's pain, alongside an appropriate pain assessment tool, you are now able to work with Angela to plan and implement an effective plan of care.

Planning and implementing pain management in LTCs

Recognising the concept of 'total pain' and the factors that influence a person's pain it is important to realise that there are many methods that can be implemented to manage pain in LTCs. These range from medication, both prescribed and over-the-counter, the use of physiotherapy and psychological care. The methods used will differ depending on the person and the type of pain being experienced. In the case of musculoskeletal pain, the management may focus on physiotherapy, relaxation and medication. The management of neuropathic pain may consist of physiotherapy, for advice regarding posture and positioning, the use of antidepressant and anticonvulsant medication and relaxation (Taverner, 2014). It may not be possible to achieve complete pain relief for everyone; if this is the case, the aim will be to reduce the pain to a level that is tolerable for the person.

Case study: Angela

Angela's pain assessment revealed that she was experiencing musculoskeletal pain, radiating down her right calf and into her foot, on six nights out of seven and occasionally during the day on four out of seven days. Angela scored her pain as being seven out of ten and described it as 'aching'; she was aware this was disturbing her usual sleep pattern and was concerned that this would increase her fatigue. The aim of the plan of care agreed between Angela and her MS CNS was to reduce both the frequency (to three out of seven nights and two out of seven days) and intensity (to four) of Angela's pain as well as to improve the quality of her sleep. Following consultation they agreed a plan of care, as follows.

Physiotherapy
The MS CNS will refer Angela to the community physiotherapist for an assessment and a planned programme of stretching exercises to help lengthen Angela's calf muscles to reduce spasm and spasticity. Physiotherapy has been shown to improve mobility in people with MS; focusing on quality of life and not just pain is known to have a positive effect (Lalkhen et al., 2012). These exercises will need to be carried out on a daily basis and Angela has agreed to write up an action plan (see Chapter 4) to ensure she is able to do this. The MS CNS has also asked that the physiotherapist consider using transcutaneous electrical nerve stimulation (TENS) as a non-pharmacological means of managing Angela's pain. The evidence surrounding TENS is varied; however it is used in the management of pain in a variety of situations. TENS stimulates the nervous system through the use of transcutaneous electrodes; this stimulation is thought to reduce the transmission of pain signals to the brain, altering the person's perception of their pain.

Relaxation
The CNS has suggested to Angela that she try relaxation as part of her ongoing pain management. Angela might find this particularly useful at night to improve the quality of her sleep. A simple technique that Angela could use would be relaxed breathing; focusing on her breathing has the potential to break the cycle of pain and anxiety by providing the mind with something else to focus on.

Prescribed medication
As a qualified nurse/independent prescriber, Angela's MS CNS is able to prescribe any licensed medication, within the sphere of her clinical competence (RCN, 2010). Based on her assessment of Angela and her pain she has prescribed an initial dose of Baclofen: 5 mg, three times a day. This can be gradually increased depending on the degree of relief Angela is experiencing. By reducing the transmission of electrical impulse along the nerves in Angela's central nervous system Baclofen will cause Angela's muscles to relax, reducing the amount of spasm and pain. As well as outlining to Angela how Baclofen works, the MS CNS has provided Angela with information regarding some of the common side-effects:

- *gastrointestinal upset: Angela has been advised to take her Baclofen after eating food and in case of nausea to eat little and often;*
- *dry mouth: chewing sugar-free gum or sweets can help reduce Angela's dry mouth;*
- *drowsiness: before driving Angela should make sure her reaction time is normal – alcohol should be avoided as it may increase her drowsiness;*
- *dizziness: getting up from either lying or sitting slowly – if the feeling continues Angela could lie down for a few minutes until the dizziness passes.*

> The MS CNS has also advised Angela that if she is concerned regarding any aspect of this medication to contact her and not to stop taking it suddenly as sudden withdrawal can cause severe side-effects. The MS CNS will visit Angela weekly over the next six weeks to review the benefits of the treatment.
>
> ### Over-the-counter medication
>
> As well as taking her prescribed medication Angela may also be taking over-the-counter medication to help manage her pain, e.g., paracetamol or ibuprofen. If this is the case it is important that the MS CNS identifies this as it is known that ibuprofen reduces the rate at which Baclofen is excreted from the body, resulting in an increased risk of toxicity. Therefore Angela should be advised to use paracetamol in preference to ibuprofen.
>
> Both Angela and the MS CNS agreed that Angela should continue to assess her musculoskeletal pain on a regular basis and devise her own action plan (Chapter 4) to identify when and how this will be done. The effectiveness of the above plan of care will be rechecked against Angela's initial pain assessment and her ongoing assessment of her musculoskeletal pain. This recheck will allow specific information, such as Angela's assessment of her pain, to be linked to the plan of care that was implemented. In the initial stages this recheck will be done on a weekly basis for the next four weeks, providing ongoing support for Angela. A formal evaluation would take place at the end of four weeks.
>
> It was decided not to refer Angela to an occupational therapist regarding splinting at this stage but to evaluate the above plan of care and refer if there was no improvement in Angela's spasm and pain.

As you can see Angela and her MS CNS worked collaboratively to compile the above plan of care. Empowerment was maintained by incorporating action planning, enabling Angela to fit her physiotherapy and pain assessment into her daily routine. Recognising the potential benefits of relaxation as a strategy Angela could use in a variety of situations will positively reflect on her QoL. The role of the MS CNS was to provide specialist knowledge regarding the pharmacological management of Angela's spasms and associated musculoskeletal pain and to refer to other members of the multidisciplinary team to maximise Angela's pain relief.

Evaluating pain management in LTCs

Evaluating the care implemented is the final stage of well-organised nursing care: the process of evaluation allows you to understand whether the care implemented has been successful in meeting the person's identified needs. Evaluating the care implemented requires a collaborative approach and should be based on how well the aims of the care have been met. Evaluating care requires you to be able to analyse all stages of the planning and implementation processes, e.g., was the pain assessment tool used appropriate, was the stated aim achievable and were the planned interventions suitable for the person and their needs (Barrett et al., 2009). By breaking the process down into its component parts, you are able to evaluate which parts were successful and which parts were not. Evaluating your care and management in this way allows you to reflect on your practice, prompting both personal and professional development.

> ## Case study: Angela
>
> *Four weeks after your initial visit to Angela with her MS CNS both you and the MS CNS are visiting Angela to evaluate the plan of care that was implemented. Angela has continued to assess her pain as outlined in her action plan; she is now experiencing pain on four nights out of seven and on two days out of seven, with her pain intensity having reduced to between three and four. She also reports that while she is still experiencing pain on four nights out of seven the quality of her sleep has improved.*
>
> ### Physiotherapy
> *Angela has found the physiotherapy to be very beneficial and has worked hard to ensure she carries out her exercises every day. As well as exercising her right leg she has been doing the same exercises with her left leg and has noticed a reduction in the severity of the muscle spasms. Angela feels this has contributed the most in reducing her musculoskeletal pain. She has not had any TENS yet, though this has been recommended by the physiotherapist.*
>
> ### Relaxation
> *Angela finds this beneficial, especially in managing her levels of stress and improving the quality of her sleep. Despite being awake due to her pain she is able to remain calm and relaxed, increasing the chances of her being able to get back to sleep.*
>
> ### Prescribed medication
> *Angela continues to take 5 mg of Baclofen three times a day; she did experience some side-effects when she initially started taking the Baclofen, mainly nausea and some dizziness. However, she is able to manage these. Despite still experiencing pain on four out of seven nights she is not keen to increase her dose of Baclofen yet.*
>
> ### Over-the-counter medication
> *Angela has not been taking any regular over-the-counter analgesics.*
>
> *Following the evaluation of the care implemented against the original aims of the care, both Angela and her MS CNS note that while the severity of Angela's pain has reduced and the quality of her sleep has improved she is still experiencing pain on four nights out of seven. As Angela is not keen to increase the dose of her Baclofen her MS CNS suggests that she asks her physiotherapist about using TENS at night. Angela agrees to this suggestion and will discuss it with her physiotherapist at her next appointment. A further recheck meeting is planned for one week's time.*

In this case study the aims of the initial plan of care were not fully met, demonstrating the cyclical nature of effective care planning and implementation. During the process of evaluation not only do you evaluate the care that has been delivered to date, you also undertake an assessment of the person's new baseline. This then leads into the planning, implementation and evaluation of further interventions.

Activity 5.5   *Decision-making*

Revisit previous chapters, pages 11 and 55, and re-read Linda's case study.

Linda is becoming more anxious; she does not go out on her own at all now and is relying on her son more frequently. She is frustrated by her situation and would like to feel more confident about herself and her health. Linda has come in to see the practice nurse at her GP surgery to talk about her situation. You are spending the day with the practice nurse and sit in on her consultation with Linda.

What plan of care could you implement to address Linda's anxiety and what members of the multidisciplinary team could you involve?

A brief outline answer is given at the end of the chapter.

As you will have seen from the scenarios above and Activity 5.5, the symptoms experienced by people living with an LTC can be multifactorial and can affect many aspects of their day-to-day life. Having an understanding of the common signs and symptoms of specific LTCs and how they are managed will assist you in your delivery of appropriate and effective symptom management.

Chapter summary

This chapter has provided you with an overview of QoL in people living with an LTC and the role that effective symptom management has in promoting and enhancing QoL. By relating effective planning of care to symptom management it has emphasised the importance of person-centred care in the effective management of symptoms in people living with an LTC.

Having read through this chapter and worked through the activities, you will have developed your knowledge and skills in relation to symptom management in the care and management of people living with an LTC. How you use this new knowledge and skills will depend on where you are working and your roles and responsibilities. However, as a nurse you can improve the care you provide to people living with an LTC, and their carers, by recognising the importance of maintaining QoL and the factors that influence QoL. By using the being, belonging and becoming model you will be able to provide holistic symptom management for those in your care. Using an effective framework for planning care, to work collaboratively with those living with an LTC, will ensure that the care and management you provide is based on a good assessment of the person's needs and is clearly focused on addressing those needs. It will also encourage you to reflect on your practice, further developing your knowledge and skills in relation to many aspects of person-centred care.

Activities: brief outline answers

Activity 5.1 Evidence-based practice and research (page 93)

COPD

COPD is an umbrella term for conditions of the respiratory system characterised by airflow obstruction; this is usually progressive and worsens over time, and includes chronic bronchitis and emphysema. COPD is characterised by the following symptoms: a cough that does not go away, regular production of sputum and breathlessness when carrying out activities (CKS, 2010). People with COPD may also experience tiredness and weight loss. Some of the physical signs that you may notice include wheeze, use of accessory muscle and peripheral oedema (CKS, 2010).

In chronic bronchitis, increased mucus production and damage to the cilia in the bronchi result in the bronchi becoming blocked with mucus. This stimulates the airway's irritant response producing a chronic cough. It is this chronic irritation that causes inflammation and thickening of the bronchial walls, which results in the airways becoming obstructed. With the cilia damaged, and not able to clear the mucus, mucus collects and blocks the smaller airways (Muralitharan and Peate, 2013). In emphysema, destruction of the alveolar wall, in the terminal bronchioles, results in enlargement of the airspaces. It is thought that the enzyme protease destroys the elastic fibres in the lungs which are needed for exhalation; this results in the alveoli becoming overinflated with air being trapped (Muralitharan and Peate, 2013). This means that there is less surface area available in the lungs for gaseous exchange to take place.

Smoking is known to be a risk factor in both chronic bronchitis and emphysema; therefore exploring smoking cessation is key in the care and management of people living with COPD. It is necessary to ensure that any prescribed inhalers (beta-2 agonists etc.) are being taken correctly; you may need to provide support regarding correct inhaler technique. In addition advice about self-management techniques to reduce breathlessness are useful, e.g., pursed lip breathing.

Type 2 diabetes

Type 2 diabetes is caused due to insulin resistance and reduced ability of beta cells in the pancreas to produce insulin. The resulting high blood glucose levels lead to further damage of the beta cells resulting in a further reduction in the production of insulin (Muralitharan and Peate, 2013). Type 2 diabetes can remain undiagnosed for some time due to the fact that the degree of hyperglycaemia is not severe enough to produce symptoms. Some common symptoms include: increased thirst, blurred vision, weight loss and lethargy (CKS, 2015).

Modifiable risk factors for type 2 diabetes include lack of exercise, obesity and smoking; therefore health education/promotion around lifestyle changes should form part of the ongoing care and management. This should include dietary advice regarding carbohydrate intake. Once a person has been diagnosed and commenced on medication to control their blood glucose level, then ongoing monitoring of their HbA_{1c} should take place to ensure this is within agreed levels. Information regarding complications should be provided, especially in relation to foot and eye care with annual reviews taking place (CKS, 2015).

Cardiovascular disease (CVD)

CVD is an umbrella term that covers any disease that involves the heart, blood vessels or both and is caused by atherosclerosis. Atherosclerosis develops when atheroma form plaques on the lining of arteries; atheroma are a complex mixture of white blood cells, lipids and calcium. Over time these plaques increase in size causing narrowing of the arteries resulting in reduced blood flow and hypertension (CKS, 2014d). Due to the nature of CVD people may experience many different symptoms, including those of angina, chest pain that may radiate to the left arm, jaw and neck, and stroke, which could include limb weakness, difficulty in speaking and facial weakness.

There are a number of known risk factors for CVD, which include smoking, lack of physical activity, increased alcohol consumption and being overweight. Advice should be given regarding smoking cessation, reducing the amount of saturated fat and increasing the amount of fish and fruit and vegetables in their diet to help reduce cholesterol, as well as taking regular exercise. It is important to ensure that any prescribed medication (e.g., statins, beta blockers) are taken as prescribed (CKS, 2014d).

Activity 5.2 Decision-making (page 97)

Domain	Sub-domain	Items included in domain and sub-domain	Areas to consider
Being: concerned with who a person is	Physical	• Physical health • Personal hygiene • Nutrition • Exercise • Grooming and clothing • General physical appearance	Due to his continence problems Joseph may be more aware of his personal hygiene requirements and take more care with these.
	Psychological	• Psychological health and adjustment • Cognition • Feelings • Self-esteem and self-control	Joseph may have low self-esteem due to his continence issues; while he realises how lucky he is, he is worried that his cancer may return.
	Spiritual	• Personal values • Personal standards of conduct • Spiritual beliefs	Joseph is an active member of his local church; this will provide both him and Grace with a sense of belonging.
Belonging: the connections a person has with their environment	Physical	• Home • Workplace/school • Neighbourhood • Community	Joseph is able to be part of his local community and is an active member of their church community.
	Social	• Intimate others • Family • Friends • Work colleagues • Neighbourhood and community	Joseph is married and has two children who live locally and who Joseph enjoys spending time with. His continence problems may affect how intimate he feels he can be with Grace.
	Community	• Adequate income • Health and social services • Employment • Education programmes • Recreation programmes • Community events and activities	Joseph and Grace are both retired, they enjoy walking and Joseph enjoys fishing – they like to keep fit and healthy. However Joseph may feel that he cannot be away from a toilet for long periods of time due to his continence problems.
Becoming: achieving goals, hopes and aspirations	Practical	• Domestic activities • Employment • School or volunteer activities • Seeing to health and social needs	Joseph is still able to look after and play with his grandchildren; he is still active and enjoys his social activities.

(Continued)

(Continued)

Domain	Sub-domain	Items included in domain and sub-domain	Areas to consider
	Leisure	• Activities that promote relaxation and reduce stress	Joseph is still able to attend church and enjoy his hobbies, though he may reduce the amount of time he spends on these due to concerns about his continence problems.
	Growth	• Activities that promote maintenance or improvement of knowledge and skills • Adapting to change	Joseph is adapting to living with cancer as a long term condition; this is causing him some anxiety as he is concerned that it may recur.

Activity 5.3 Critical thinking (page 99)

How do we feel pain?

There are pain receptors (nociceptors) within our skin, periosteum, arterial walls, joint surfaces and the lining of our cranium. Damage to these tissues stimulates local pain receptors, allowing pain to be easily localised and identified, for example a person with osteoarthritis who has pain in their knees. Pain receptors in other parts of the body, mainly the organs, are supplied by a larger, more diffuse arrangement of pain receptors. This may make locating pain more difficult as the pain can be experienced over a larger area. There are some organs in the body where there are almost no pain receptors, e.g. the liver parenchyma and the alveoli in the lungs. However, the liver capsule, the bronchi and parietal pleura are very sensitive to pain. Pain receptors are free nerve endings that are activated by stimuli such as pressure (mechanoreceptors), extremes of temperature (thermoreceptors) and chemical substances (chemoreceptors) (Porth and Matfin, 2010). Chronic pain is felt due to the fact that pain receptors do not adapt to sustained stimulation but keep on being activated and producing signals. This is because the body's natural analgesics need to be stimulated to remind the person to protect that area of their body to help manage the pain. Acute and chronic pain sensations are transmitted via sensory nerves to the thalamus and hypothalamus. Acute pain sensations are transmitted via larger A-delta fibres that are able to carry a larger number of impulses while chronic pain sensations are transmitted via smaller C fibres carrying a lower number of impulses (Porth and Matfin, 2010).

What is the difference between nociceptive and neuropathic pain?

Nociceptive pain is pain that is felt due to the activation of pain receptors (nociceptors). This type of pain is usually due to tissue damage, e.g. trauma, surgery or disease progression. It is often described as sharp, aching, crushing or throbbing. Neuropathic pain is felt when the nerve itself is damaged by compression or infiltration; the damaged nerve then sends signals to the rest of the nervous system. Due to damage to the sensory nerves the pain may be experienced in an area where there is numbness. Neuropathic pain is often described as burning, stabbing or like pins and needles (Porth and Matfin, 2010). An example of this is shingles (herpes zoster infection); this can cause peripheral neuropathic pain. This pain is often described as hot, burning, stabbing, shooting or tingling.

What are the body's natural analgesics?

The body's natural analgesics are opioid peptides (dynophorins and endorphins) produced in the hypothalamus and pituitary gland that are found in the nervous system in the areas of the brain associated with pain reception. They are also found in areas of the spinal cord. Their distribution corresponds to the areas of the brain where electrical stimulation can control pain, such as the thalamus. When a person experiences pain these opioid peptides are released at the point where the pain signal enters the spinal cord and at the synapses in the thalamus, hypothalamus and cerebral cortex (Porth and Matfin, 2010).

Activity 5.4 Evidence-based practice and research (page 102)

Aspects	Influencing factors	Application to practice
Physical	The condition The person's functional capacity Side-effects of treatment Disfigurement	Angela may realise that this symptom could be permanent and that she may experience further deteriorations in her functional capacity. Her disturbed sleep may be a contributing factor.
Social	Family issues Loss of role at work Loss of role at home Finances Change in appearance due to condition Sense of helplessness	Angela is currently off work; depending on her illness benefits this may have a financial impact on her and her family. In addition she may feel she is not able to fulfill her role as a mother.
Spiritual	Purpose Religion Meaning Uncertainty about future Hope Fear of pain/death	This relapse may be a reminder to Angela of the ongoing nature of her RRMS and that it will become progressively worse.
Psychological	Anger Delays in diagnosis Coping ability Control and sense of usefulness Failure of treatment	Angela may question her ability to cope with her condition; she may be concerned that as her condition worsens she may become a 'burden'.

Some methods of pain assessment:

- taking a pain history – assessing the site, nature and duration of the pain as well as factors that relieve and exacerbate it;
- physical examination – may help confirm the cause of the pain; will also allow examination of other aspects, such as nutrition;
- body charts – pictures of the human body where the person can indicate and record the location of any pain; these can be updated;
- numerical and visual analogue scales – includes 0–3 and 0–10 numerical scale and the no pain to worse pain or no pain relief to complete pain relief visual analogue scale;
- picture scales – use of faces with expressions ranging from happiness to distress;
- pain questionnaires and inventories – these question the person on a range of factors relating to their pain, e.g., pain intensity, mood, pain relief.

Using communication skills, such as active listening, touch and observation, and engaging in a therapeutic relationship with Angela, will enhance the assessment process, enabling you and Angela to work together to manage her pain.

Activity 5.5 Decision-making (page 107)

The aim of your plan would be to increase Linda's coping strategies to reduce her anxiety and increase her confidence. To do this you would need to undertake a holistic assessment of Linda and try to identify the trigger for her anxiety; this could be related to the sudden and unexpected nature of her husband's death.

You would want to recheck Linda's progress, and the suitability of your plan, weekly with a formal evaluation being arranged in approximately four weeks' time.

Using an action plan would be an appropriate way to ensure that Linda was in control of her care; however due to her lack of confidence you may need to work with her to compile this. The goal of Linda's action plan could be that she goes outside to her garden by herself; you would need to ensure that Linda's confidence level in achieving this is above 7 to make it a realistic goal for her to achieve. You could incorporate relaxation into Linda's action plan, e.g., focused breathing and relaxation could reduce her anxiety but in addition it could help manage her breathlessness. Initially you may not involve other members of the multidisciplinary team in Linda's care, however you may discuss her anxiety with her GP, heart failure CNS or community based occupational therapist. Depending on whether there is an improvement in Linda's anxiety or not you may need to refer on to more specialist support, such as cognitive behavioural therapy.

Further reading

Chatterjee, J (2012) Improving pain assessment for patients with cognitive impairment: development of a pain assessment toolkit. *International Journal of Palliative Care,* 18 (12): 581–9.

This article describes how a pain assessment toolkit was developed to support individualised pain assessment for people with a cognitive impairment

Osborne, LA, Bindemann, N, Noble, JG and Reed, P (2012) Changes in the key areas of quality of life associated with age and time since diagnosis of long-term conditions. *Chronic Illness,* 8 (2): 112–20.

This research article investigated the relationship between QoL, age and time since diagnosis. Results showed that the areas people feel important change over time; this has implications for how QoL might be assessed.

Shah, C, Lehman, H and Richardson, S (2014) Medicines optimisation: an agenda for community nursing. *Journal of Community Nursing,* 28 (3): 82–5.

Useful website

http://cks.nice.org.uk/#?char=A

The homepage of Clinical Knowledge Summaries: a useful, evidence-based resource providing information about the care and management of a range of LTCs.

Chapter 6
Managing complex care in long term conditions

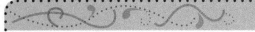

NMC Essential Skills Clusters

Cluster: Organisational aspects of care

This chapter will address the following ESCs:

13. People can trust the newly registered graduate nurse to promote continuity when their care is to be transferred to another service or person.

By the second progression point:

1. Assists in preparing people and carers for transfer and transition through effective dialogue and accurate information.
2. Reports issues and people's concerns regarding transfer and transition.
3. Assists in the preparation of records and reports to facilitate safe and effective transfer.

Chapter aims

After reading this chapter you will be able to:

- understand the role case management has in the management of people with LTCs who have complex care needs;
- explain the roles and responsibilities of the case manager in the care of people living with an LTC;
- use care pathways to support person-centred care for those living with an LTC who have complex needs;
- recognise the importance of effective discharge planning for people living with an LTC and their carers.

Introduction

Delivering improvements for people with long term conditions isn't about just treating illness, it's about delivering personalised, responsive, holistic care in the full context of how people want to live their lives.

(DH, 2008, p. 5)

The ageing population of the UK means that by 2025 the number of people over the age of 65 will increase by 42% resulting in an associated increase in the incidence of LTCs. While it is recognised that people living with one or more LTCs are intensive users of health and social care services, it is also known that increasing a person's sense of self-worth promotes their desire to manage their own health (DH, 2008). The majority of people living with LTCs will have their condition managed effectively through appropriate health promotion and health education, self-management and timely symptom management. However, some people living with multiple LTCs will have more complex health and social care needs. This group of people, for a variety of reasons, e.g. living with multiple LTCs, multiple episodes of unplanned hospital admissions or living on their own, are likely to experience a reduced QoL. They require a range of integrated services, and the delivery of proactive care and management which is coordinated by a suitably qualified person.

Case study: Andrew

Andrew is a 76-year-old widower and is living with chronic obstructive pulmonary disease (COPD).

Andrew lives alone in a one-bedroomed flat in a sheltered housing complex.

Over the last 12 months Andrew has been experiencing worsening health, and has had two admissions to hospital, for chest infections, in the last three months. This is despite his district nurse working with Andrew to increase his level of exercise and improve his nutritional intake. After some initial success Andrew was not able to maintain his level of exercise and due to his increasing dyspnoea he has been relying on meals on wheels to provide him with a hot meal. His recent chest infections have left him with worsening dyspnoea and associated reduction in his mobility. Care workers visit twice a day to assist Andrew with washing and dressing, and a neighbour pops in to dust, vacuum and help with his laundry. At the weekly practice meeting, following his last admission, his GP has transferred Andrew's care over to the community matron for case management.

David will be Andrew's case manager; David is a qualified district nurse and, working as part of the practice team, will be responsible for coordinating Andrew's care and management. David will use a case management approach to ensure that Andrew's ongoing physical, social and psychological needs are met. By leading, and taking responsibility for, Andrew's care David will coordinate input from other agencies, ensuring that Andrew's care needs are met. Through working with Andrew, and as his single point of contact, David will support Andrew to make informed choices about the care he receives. David will further work with Andrew to encourage him to be aware of changes in his condition that signal an exacerbation and to take action to address these.

Andrew's story demonstrates that the aim of case management is to streamline the care and management of complex needs that result from living with multiple LTCs. You may not be directly involved in the case management of people living with LTCs, though it may be that, when working with a community matron or specialist respiratory nurse, you observe the management of complex care needs for this group of people. Integrating the knowledge from previous chapters in relation to health promotion and health education, self-management and symptom management will enable you to assist in the delivery of effective case management and complex care. To further support you in your role this chapter will develop your knowledge and understanding of case management and complex care. In order to do this the chapter will discuss the roles and responsibilities of case managers and how the care of those requiring complex care is managed. The chapter also discusses the way in which care pathways can be used and examines the importance of discharge planning for those living with LTCs who have been admitted to secondary care.

Case management in LTCs

Case management originated in the USA where, in the 1950s, it was used as a means of providing care to people with severe mental health needs. From this it was then rolled out and used with older people who had complex health and social care needs. The aim of case management is to provide care that is personalised and responsive to the changing needs of people living with LTCs, promoting QoL and reducing the need for long term care (Bentley, 2014). In the UK case management has been used in mental health nursing since the 1980s; this was as a response to the shift from institutionalised to community care. Since then it has formed part of the care and management of people living with LTCs. As well as streamlining the care provided, the aim of case management is to enable people living with LTCs who require complex care to stay at home for longer and to have more choice about their care.

Activity 6.1   *Reflection*

Case management is a key part of the care and management of people living with an LTC. On your own or with a group of colleagues, reflect on the areas where you have undertaken clinical practice and consider the following questions.

- What members of the health and social care team undertake the role of case manager?
- What are their roles and responsibilities in relation to managing the care of people with LTCs?
- How do they fit in with other health and social care professionals?

As the answers will be based on your own observations there is no outline answer at the end of this chapter.

Undertaking Activity 6.1 will have shown you that case management can be undertaken by a range of health and social care professionals. These may include district nurses, nurse specialists and community matrons, physiotherapists and social workers.

Roles and responsibilities of the case manager in LTCs

In completing Activity 6.1 you will have begun to identify some of the roles and responsibilities case managers have; case managers have both strategic and patient-focused responsibilities. In the literature the terms case manager and community matron are used interchangeably, and there is some overlapping of roles. Generally speaking: case managers are responsible for coordinating the care and management of people living with LTCs who have a complex single LTC or social need. They will be responsible for planning, monitoring and anticipating the needs of those living with one or more LTCs. In this situation the case manager is likely to be a qualified nurse, social worker or other healthcare professional. Community matrons are responsible for supporting high intensity patients who require the input of advanced clinical skills (such as advanced health assessment) and clinical management as in, for example, management of hydration (Bentley, 2014).

Whereas the level of clinical nursing care may vary between case managers and community matrons, the roles and responsibilities of the case manager or community matron should be underpinned by the following core elements (Bentley, 2014):

- case finding or screening to identify suitable patients;
- person-centred assessment and diagnosis;
- holistic care planning and implementation of care;
- referral of patient to appropriate services and coordination of these;
- monitoring and evaluation of services and patient outcomes, e.g., independence maintained.

It is the responsibility of the case manager/community matron to ensure that the core elements listed above form the basis of their roles and responsibilities in relation to people living with an LTC. Using Andrew's case scenario, Table 6.1 provides you with some points to consider and applies these core elements to clinical practice.

Core elements	Points to consider	Application to practice
Case finding or screening	Identifying people, through the use of referral criteria, who may benefit from a case management approach. Be aware of hidden populations, e.g. homeless, asylum seekers and travellers. Some examples of referral criteria include: • must be over 18 years of age; • people who frequently use health/social care services; • people who have had two or more accident and emergency and/or hospital admissions in the past 12 months; • people who have one or more LTC; • people who are taking four or more medications.	Andrew has had two unplanned hospital admissions in the last three months. When at home he has a care package for assistance with his personal hygiene and a neighbour cooks meals and helps with housework. His current health status means that he is eligible for a case management approach to his care and management.

(Continued)

Table 6.1 (Continued)

Core elements	Points to consider	Application to practice
Assessment	Assessing a person's health and social care needs using recognised assessments. Using information gathered from the person, their carer and family and other services involved in the person's care. Be aware of obtaining consent to share information and confidentiality. This may include undertaking a physical health assessment, making a diagnosis and non-medical prescribing.	Working with Andrew, David will assess his current health and social care needs, including his concordance and compliance with his medication regime. Given Andrew's current health status this is likely to include a physical health assessment. David will review the current level of support to ensure it is meeting Andrew's health and social care needs. Areas highlighted in David's assessment may include improving his nutritional intake and educating Andrew about the signs that indicate his condition is deteriorating.
Care planning	Formulating a personalised care plan to meet the needs identified in the assessment. This care plan may also address anticipated needs. If required, the care plan is agreed with the person's GP and consultant. Coordinates input from other members of the health and social care team who may also have some clinical input.	This will depend on the result of Andrew's assessment; it will be David's responsibility to coordinate the input of other agencies. David may refer Andrew on for further nutritional support; David may be required to prescribe nutritional supplements. David is also likely to provide Andrew with information regarding his condition.
Implementation of care plan	Maintaining contact with the person and monitoring input from other health and social care professionals. Provides clinical care if required.	David will become Andrew's single point of contact; he will remain visible to Andrew, ensuring that the care plan is well coordinated. David may also undertake ongoing monitoring of Andrew's physical health status.
Monitoring and reviewing	Monitoring the effectiveness of the care plan and reviewing the level of care if required. Using care pathways and protocols to streamline care.	David will review Andrew's care plan on a regular basis, depending on his current health status. David may use care pathways to support Andrew's care, e.g. acute exacerbation of COPD care pathway.

Table 6.1: Application of the core elements of case management (as described by Offredy, 2009) to your clinical practice

As you can see from Table 6.1, the core elements of case management allow David, as Andrew's community matron, to coordinate and guide his care. Ensuring a single point of contact will improve communication between all health and social care professionals involved in Andrew's care, and with Andrew himself.

Research summary

A literature review carried out by Sutherland and Hayter (2009) focused on the effectiveness of case management as undertaken by nurses in improving health outcomes in the following LTCs: diabetes, COPD and coronary heart disease. Only studies that evaluated case management with one or all of the three LTCs identified were included in the review. A thematic analysis of the literature was carried out using the health outcomes that were appraised in the chosen articles. Sutherland and Hayter (2009) found that case management was effective in improving a person's level of self-care and increasing their level of psychosocial support. In addition, through effective assessment and monitoring, the progression of their LTC was managed more effectively. They concluded that case management has the potential to improve health outcomes for people living with LTCs, however they expressed the need for further research to be carried out to support the development of a more targeted approach to care (Sutherland and Hayter, 2009).

Research in 2014 by Randall et al. explored case management in relation to support for people living with a range of LTCs. This mixed methodology quantitative study used a combination of focus groups (with case managers), audio diaries (case managers) and semi-structured interviews (with case managers, patients and their carers and secondary care staff) to explore all aspects of case management. To provide consistency of data analysis the domains of case management (NHS Modernisation Agency and Skills for Health, 2005) were used. The findings identified the following themes:

- Visibility – knowing that the case manager was there and how to contact her was important to both patients and carers. Secondary care staff valued the input of the case manager, especially in relation to knowing and understanding the home environment of the patient. In contrast case managers felt that their role was not understood by secondary care staff.
- Interpersonal relationships – for patients and their carers being seen as an individual was valued; having a trusting relationship with their case manager improved the patients' mental wellbeing and provided an additional layer of support. Case managers identified the central role of this relationship as promoting and enabling self-care and management, reducing access to secondary care services.
- Leadership – case managers found it challenging to separate out leadership and management, though they were clearer about their role in the coordination of care and taking a leadership role in directing the wider healthcare team.

(Continued)

(Continued)

- System and professional boundaries – secondary care staff reported confusion in understanding the role of the case manager; this was in part due to organisational boundaries meaning that secondary care staff had contact with three separate community trusts. Difficulty in accessing out of hours care was mentioned by patients, their carers and the case managers, with advice often being to contact emergency services.

As you can see from the above research summary case management has a positive effect on people living with LTCs and their family and carers, particularly in relation to support and coordination of care.

Activity 6.2 — *Reflection*

Reflecting back on your recent clinical experience identify a person, living with LTCs, who had complex care needs and compile a map or diagram of the services involved in their care and management.

Using the information provided in Table 6.1, apply the core elements to your chosen person and review how case management could have improved their care and management.

As the answers will be based on your own observations there is no outline answer at the end of this chapter.

As discussed above, Activity 6.2 will have demonstrated to you how, through ensuring an appropriate and responsive plan of care is in place, case management can be used to improve the care and management of people living with LTCs. In your current role you may not be actively involved in case management; however, using the information in Table 6.1 in your nursing practice will support you in your delivery of effective care to people living with LTCs.

Managing complex care

For some people living with LTCs it is inevitable that as their condition deteriorates their health and social care needs will become increasingly more complex. One group of people who fall into this category, who have not been mentioned previously, are those living with frailty. It is generally recognised that the majority of LTCs affect a specific physiological system (e.g., cardiovascular, endocrine), or a specific organ (e.g. lung cancer, COPD), and that as the disease progresses symptoms will increase as will the level of care and management they require. Increasingly, alongside this more traditional view of LTCs, frailty is being recognised as an LTC.

Frailty as an LTC

'The frail elderly' is a term that is often used to describe a group of people, such as those who are dependent on others for their ADLs, rather than being seen as a diagnosed medical condition. Like other LTCs frailty is progressive, has a negative impact on health and wellbeing and can result in people becoming acutely unwell if not managed carefully. It is estimated that approximately 10% of people over the age of 65 have frailty. This rises to between 25–50% of those over the age of 85 (Clegg et al., 2013). Frailty is not an illness but a syndrome that is related to the ageing process; in frailty multiple body systems gradually lose their reserves. Its aetiology is not fully understood but it is thought that changes in a person's immune system and a decline in musculoskeletal and endocrine systems are involved (Chen et al., 2014), resulting in a gradual decline in physical and cognitive function. Recognising frailty is not easy; older people may not see themselves as being 'frail'. They may have made adjustments in their daily activities over time and are not aware of how 'frail' they are. It may not be until an acute event, such as a fall or a chest infection, that a person's level of 'frailty' is identified.

To support the identification, care and management of frailty, the British Geriatric Society (BGS) in 2014 published *Fit for Frailty: Consensus best practice guidance for the care of older people living with frailty in community and outpatient settings*. The BGS (2014) identifies five syndromes that could indicate a person has frailty. These are: falls, immobility, delirium, incontinence and susceptibility to side-effects of medication. If you are caring for a person presenting with any of these syndromes then this is an opportunity for you to identify if a person is frail. There is a range of tests that you can use including the *timed up and go test*. This measures, in seconds, how long it takes a person to stand up from a standard chair, walk a distance of up to 3 metres, turn, walk back and sit down. The cut off time for this test is 10 seconds (BGS, 2014). This test is easy to carry out and requires no specific equipment making it ideal to carry out in a range of settings. Once a person

Clinical concern	Practical interventions
Under-nutrition	Refer to dietitian for assessment and nutritional support; provide education regarding what foods to eat – should include high energy and high protein foods. If person is in a hospital setting use of red tray system and provide assistance at meal times.
Challenging behaviour (delirium)	Identify if there is an underlying cause: pain, constipation or urinary retention and investigate. Be alert to changes in the person's attitude that could indicate they are becoming agitated, e.g. facial expressions, verbal threats. Use of de-escalation techniques, such as asking open questions, listening and paying attention to the person.
Reduced mobility	Refer to physiotherapy for strengthening and balance exercises, ideally for 2 hours per week, to reduce the incidence of falls. Ensure the environment is uncluttered with any trip hazards removed. Encourage correct use of mobility aids.

Table 6.2: Interventions to manage aspects of frailty

has been diagnosed with frailty it is important to manage this and maintain the person's overall health and well-being; some examples of this are provided in Table 6.2.

As you can see from Table 6.2 there are some very practical steps that you can use to manage frailty, maintaining quality of life for the person. For those involved in caring for people with frailty, and other LTCs, there are some useful resources available to support them in their delivery of person-centred care. One such resource is integrated care pathways (ICPs). ICPs are also known as care pathways and maps of care, but for consistency the term integrated care pathway (ICP) will be used in this chapter.

Integrated care pathways and LTCs

An integrated care pathway (ICP) is a framework that allows an interprofessional approach to care; its aim is to support a person, with a specific condition, or set of symptoms, to move through health and social care services. The aim of ICPs is to improve both the coordination and consistency of care a person receives. They allow you to *deliver the right care to the right person in the right place and at the right time.* ICPs can be used in different ways.

They can be used to promote equity of care across a range of care settings by providing clear guidance and advice regarding the steps to be taken when providing care to a specific group of people. Examples are the integrated care pathways used for mental health in Scotland; these pathways detail the specific care of people with mental health needs. In relation to depression they provide you with guidance from the point of diagnosis, ensure that a validated assessment tool is used, through to accessing specialist treatment for recurrent and ongoing depression. The care pathway incorporates best evidence and national guidelines to support the care you provide (NHS Quality Improvement Scotland, 2007). ICPs can also be used to provide a framework for the multidisciplinary team to use for specific health or social care situations, such as acute stroke. In this instance an ICP is used as the single document that all health and social care professionals use to document the clinical care. This single point of communication has the potential to lead to improved communication and coordination of care. Using an ICP can support you to deliver interprofessional and multi-agency working and can empower patients and their carers to actively participate more in their care.

While most ICPs have a clear clinical focus, such as depression, others take a more encompassing approach such as Age UK's integrated care pathway. This pathway brings together health, social care and voluntary organisations, putting the older person in control of their health, enabling them to maintain their independence and quality of life. The aim is to have services 'wrap around' the older person; the pathway is reviewed regularly with protocols put in place should the older person's situation change (Age UK, 2014).

Activity 6.3   *Reflection*

Either on your own, or with a colleague, reflect back on the action plans, care plans and integrated care pathways you have used in your clinical practice and answer the following questions:

- How were they used to support patient care?
- Did they support interprofessional working? If so how? If not why?
- Did they support the delivery of person-centred care? If so how? If not why?
- Were they focused on a specific condition and intervention? If so was the focus of this acute or long term?

As the answers will be based on your own observations there is no outline answer at the end of this chapter.

You may have identified from Activity 6.3 that you have used a range of care planning strategies at difference times and for different reasons. It is likely however that whichever tool you used, you planned care to take into consideration a person's physical, social, psychological and spiritual health, the impact this has on their symptoms and how they manage them.

It should be noted, however, that while ICPs form the template of the care to be delivered, the people receiving the care are individuals and will not all respond in the same way and follow the same pathway of care. It is necessary therefore that these individualities are accommodated within the ICP. These individualities are known as 'variances'. Variances allow for healthcare professionals to use their professional judgement in relation to the care being delivered. Recognising and managing variances requires you, as a student nurse, to be able to problem-solve. Effective care planning, as discussed in Chapter 5, will support you in your ability to do this. When a variance is noted, the following should be recorded on the care pathway: what variance occurred and why, the action taken (personalised care plan) and the outcome of the action. The aim of the action taken in relation to a variance is to return the person to the ICP as soon as possible (Middleton et al., 2001). Table 6.3 outlines how a care planning tool such as the nursing process can be applied to ICPs and managing variances in a person's care.

The nursing process	Integrated care pathway	Application to practice
Assess	You are using an acute stroke ICP and are undertaking an initial assessment regarding the person's skin integrity.	You use a recognised risk assessment tool, e.g. the Waterlow pressure ulcer risk assessment tool, to assess the person's skin.
Systematic nursing diagnosis	This assessment gives you a risk score of 22, indicating that the person has a very high risk of developing a pressure ulcer.	
Plan	You record the result of your assessment on the initial assessment sheet, and as a variance, to ensure that all members of the healthcare team are aware of the results of your assessment. As you have recorded a variance you compile a specific care plan to address the patient's high risk score.	You develop a care plan to maintain skin integrity; this should include what the patient can do and what the MD team will do, and should include clear aims and goals. You implement the use of pressure relieving equipment and plan a range of nursing activities and other healthcare measures.

(Continued)

Table 6.3   (Continued)

The nursing process	Integrated care pathway	Application to practice
Implement	In addition to using appropriate pressure reducing equipment, working with the person you implement a care plan and set goals that address the following aspects of nursing care: • general nursing care – regular positional changes; • liaise with physiotherapist regarding positioning and mobility assessment; • pain – any pain is being assessed and well controlled; • nutrition – a high protein nutritious diet is available; • person handling – the correct moving and lifting techniques are used; • skin care – good personal hygiene, ensuring that the skin in kept clean and dry. As care is provided this is then recorded on the ICP; this may include how frequently specific aspects of care are to be delivered.	
Recheck	You record, on the ongoing assessment of the plan of care, the care planned. This will include any reassessment of the person's skin integrity using Waterlow. You record this change on the ongoing assessment of the plan of care. When providing care you notice a change in skin integrity and record on the variance analysis sheet.	There is a change in skin colour on the right heel: the skin is intact; however, **non-blanching erythema** is present. As a grade one pressure ulcer is classed as a wound you implement a care plan to address this. This includes: • regular positional changes; • ensuring that there is no pressure on the right heel; • applying a film or thin hydrocolloid dressing for protection.
Evaluate	Using the ICP, and identified care plan to address the grade one pressure ulcer, ensures that evaluation takes place as documented. This evaluation consists of: • ongoing pressure ulcer risk assessment; • ongoing review of the care plan.	

Table 6.3: Application of the nursing process and an integrated care pathway to your clinical practice

As you can see from Table 6.3, by providing you with a clear framework within which to work, both the nursing process and ICPs are useful resources to use to support your delivery of person-centred care.

Activity 6.4   *Evidence-based practice and research*

During your next practice learning experience, with the support of your mentor, find the ICPs that are used to support care; these could be local or national. Considering the following questions review a selection of these.

- Is there a clear evidence base presented for the ICP?
- Is there a regular review date?
- Is the ICP linked to other policy within the trust?
- Is there clear guidance on how to complete the ICP?
- Is the ICP easy to navigate: do you know where to document your initial assessment, ongoing care and variances?

You could include this activity as evidence in your portfolio in support of the NMC (2010) *Standards for Pre-Registration Nursing Education*, especially in relation to leadership, management and team work.

As the answers will be based on your own observations there is no outline answer at the end of this chapter.

Undertaking Activity 6.4 will have identified that ICPs not only support the delivery of responsive person-centred care, they can also be used to support the delivery of evidence-based and cost-effective health and social care. NICE provides a range of online pathways that map their guidance; these are quick and easy to use. NICE Pathways incorporate a range of conditions/situations including acute heart failure to walking and cycling. The broad breadth of the NICE Pathways allows clinicians to access evidence-based pathways to support person-centred, holistic care for those with LTCs.

Each pathway is supported by an appropriate evidence base including research and clinical guidelines; this ensures that the information provided is based on best available evidence and is suitable for use throughout the UK. While the maps are not as detailed as an ICP they do provide information regarding treatment options and where care should be delivered, e.g. in primary or secondary care.

Case study: Joseph – using NICE Pathways

It is likely that NICE Pathways guided the care and management of Joseph's prostate cancer. For example following his biopsy, once his Gleason score was known, the pathway would have indicated that Joseph's cancer was 'intermediate risk'. This result would have signposted the clinicians to offer radical treatment to Joseph, either prostatectomy or radiotherapy. Included in this pathway is how to manage any adverse effects of radical treatment, for example incontinence, which Joseph is experiencing. This pathway also includes what follow-up treatment Joseph should expect to receive.

As discussed in this chapter the effective use of case management and care pathways improves the care and management for people living with LTCs, supporting independence and reducing unnecessary admission to secondary care. However it is recognised that it is not always possible to manage all acute exacerbations in primary care and that, at times, admission to hospital is necessary. For people living with LTCs, and their carers, admission to secondary care can be a time of stress and anxiety, especially if the person has complex care needs. Hospital admission can place a person at risk of hospital-acquired infection; it can often result in a reduction in a person's functional ability, especially in older people and those with a cognitive impairment, and can increase a person's social isolation.

Research summary: Dementia and secondary care

For people with dementia, removal from their familiar surroundings where they may just be able to 'cope', to an unfamiliar setting where it is busy and there are lots of new faces, can be bewildering. It is known that up to 97% of nurses in a secondary (or tertiary) care setting are responsible for caring for people with dementia (Alzheimer's Society, 2009). In a busy ward environment people with dementia can be seen as being 'challenging' to nurses: they require more time to be spent with them, they may display unpredictable behaviour, they may wander, and communication with them can be difficult. From the perspective of the carer, findings from the Alzheimer's Society's report (2009) noted that up to 47% of carers said that admission to secondary care had a negative effect on the physical health of the individual with dementia and 54% of carers said that an admission to secondary care had a negative effect on the symptoms of dementia, for example increased confusion and changes in behaviour. It is important, therefore, both for nurses and for those with dementia, that strategies are in place to support nurses to maximise care and to ensure that for those living with dementia any deterioration in their condition is minimised. Strategies that have been identified include the following (Heath et al., 2010):

- Improving orientation to the environment – this requires a committed approach from hospital management. Improving lighting, reducing noise and providing signposting, especially to toilets, can improve a person's orientation and reduce agitation (Waller, 2012). Personalising a person's bed space and locker will enable them to identify it easily and will provide reassurance.
- Using a 'This is Me' guide and/or memory books (see Chapter 4) – these are simple and practical tools that provide an overview of the person with dementia. 'This is Me' addresses areas such as the person's ability to manage their activities of daily living, their likes and dislikes and what worries them. For information on memory books see the section on self-management for people living with dementia in Chapter 4 of this book.
- Learning from carers – as previously mentioned in this book, carers play an important role in supporting people living with an LTC, and it is important to use their knowledge of the person to inform the care you are providing. Carers may also be willing to participate in a person's care, for example, helping them to eat at meal times, though you will need to take into consideration the privacy of other patients in the ward should this happen.

- Improving communication – finding suitable ways of communication with people who have dementia will improve the quality of care given. Observing the person and talking to their carer will enable the most appropriate method to be found, for example, using pictures, and observing facial expressions and body postures. By speaking clearly, keeping language simple, using the person's name consistently and demonstrating warmth, communication can be improved and levels of understanding increased.

The strategies identified above, such as working with carers, improving communication, learning about the person and effective pain assessment and management (see Chapter 5, page 99–106) have the potential to minimise the risk of challenging behaviours occurring. However, it is acknowledged that episodes of challenging behaviour may still occur, and using the ABC approach to assess challenging behaviour can support effective management (Heath et al., 2010).

- A – Antecedents/triggers: what was happening before the challenging behaviour occurred? Who was present and where did it happen?

- B – Behaviour: what challenging behaviour occurred? Has this happened before or is this behaviour new?

- C – Consequences: what happened as a result of this behaviour?

Using the strategies outlined above will improve the care delivered to those with dementia, and their carers, while in secondary care. By working to minimise any deterioration in a person's level of cognitive ability and supporting and working with carers, appropriate and timely discharge can be achieved.

People living with LTCs who are admitted to hospital often have care packages at home that need to be reviewed or reinstated before discharge. For some people they may not have had any input prior to admission but because of a change in their health status they require care on discharge. Therefore it is important that any discharge is planned effectively and in a timely manner. Beginning to plan for discharge on admission has the potential to minimise a person's length of stay, maximising their function and minimising the risk of complications. When discharging a person with LTCs from hospital it is important that this process is planned.

Discharge planning in LTCs

Discharge should not be seen as a discreet part of a patient's care; it should be seen as an interactive process that starts on admission. However in reality it often starts when a person is deemed 'medically fit for discharge', meaning that the process can be rushed and completed in a short space of time. A Cochrane Review by Shepperd et al. (2013) found that effective discharge planning reduced overall length of stay and reduced readmission rates in older people. They also found that discharge planning increased patient, and carer, satisfaction. However it is recognised that there are many factors that influence when discharge planning starts and how effectively it is managed. In a busy acute setting the priority might be on the person's acute presentation, and managing that, rather than on starting discharge planning (Rhudy et al., 2009). The multidisciplinary nature of the care and management of people with complex care needs means that coordination of the discharge planning process can be problematic (Rhudy et al., 2009).

The important role discharge planning plays has been recognised by the NHS Institute for Innovation and Improvement (2010) in their *High Impact Actions for Nursing and Midwifery: The Essential Collection*. The High Impact Actions represent the areas of care where poor patient experience is evident, and they include:

- your skin matters;
- staying safe – preventing falls;
- keeping nourished – getting better;
- promoting normal birth;
- important choices – where to die when the time comes;
- fit and well to care;
- ready to go – no delays;
- protection from infection.

The aim of this initiative is to strengthen the role nurses can play across a range of key clinical areas. From the list above you will see that they relate to other topics discussed in previous chapters. For example 'fit and well to care', see Chapter 2. With the development of bed managers and discharge coordinators, nurses can feel disengaged from the discharge planning process; 'ready to go – no delays' promotes nurse-led discharge as a strategy to ensure people are discharged in a timely manner. At the same time *High Impact Actions for Nursing and Midwifery: The Essential Collection* (NHS Institute, 2010) was published, the DH published *Ready to Go? Planning the Discharge and the Transfer of Patients from Hospital and Intermediate Care* (DH, 2010). The 10-step framework discussed in this document can be used to support effective, nurse-led discharge.

Case study: Linda (see Chapter 3 for further information)

Linda was admitted to hospital after being found lying on the floor by her son. He was concerned when she did not answer the phone and had called round to see if she was alright. When he found Linda, she was a bit confused and the left side of her face was drooping. Linda could not remember what had happened, and was not sure how long she had been lying there for; she had tried to get herself up but was not able to. Her son phoned an ambulance and she was admitted to hospital; on admission her blood glucose levels were found to be elevated (HbA$_{1c}$ was 50 mmol/mol). Over the next 24 hours her confusion resolved as did the drooping of the left side of her face. However, Linda's blood glucose levels remained elevated after admission; a diagnosis of type 2 diabetes was made and she was commenced on metformin 500 mg twice a day (BD). Linda does not like being in hospital and is keen to get home to a familiar environment.

In Table 6.4, the DH 10-step framework has been applied to Linda's discharge planning.

Step	Key points	Application to Linda
1. Start planning for discharge on or before admission	Start discharge planning before or on admission. Undertake a full assessment. Record any factors which may make discharge problematic. Ensure MD team are aware of their roles and responsibilities. Involve carers/family.	As Linda was an emergency admission, you will have to start this on admission. Carry out a full assessment, including medication and social situation. Linda lives alone and is socially isolated due to her anxiety. Liaise with the physiotherapist regarding mobility as Linda was admitted with a suspected fall at home. With Linda's consent Linda's son should be informed about any plans for discharge.
2. Identify if the patient has simple or complex discharge planning needs	Simple discharge – person is likely to return to their own home and does not require complex ongoing care. Complex discharge – person requires complex ongoing health and/or social care input from an MD and/or interagency team.	While Linda has been diagnosed with having had a TIA and has been newly diagnosed with type 2 diabetes, she does not require complex ongoing care – therefore she has simple discharge planning needs.
3. Develop a clinical management plan within 24 hours of admission	This care plan should include treatment activities and goals, how these goals are going to be achieved and the estimated timeframe. Diagnostic and investigative treatments should also be included.	Linda has been referred to the dietitian regarding her diabetes and for advice about her diet and how to make healthy changes. Due to Linda's anxiety she may require support from the MD team regarding confidence building to support her when she is home. There has been a change to Linda's medication, therefore medicines optimisation should take place with Linda to ensure that she understands her new medication. A date is set for Linda's discharge.

(Continued)

Table 6.4   (Continued)

Step	Key points	Application to Linda
4. Coordinate the discharge through effective leadership and handover of responsibilities at ward level	Due to individual staff not being available every day, each day one person should take responsibility for coordinating the discharge planning process. Documentation should be kept up to date, both written and verbal (handover). For complex discharges discharge coordinators may manage the process.	Keep Linda's case records up to date, document her progress and whether discharge planning is on track, liaise and coordinate the input of other members of the MD team.
5. Set an expected date of discharge within 24–48 hours of admission and discuss with carer/family	This can be based on the patient's clinical picture: are they improving, staying the same or deteriorating? How long it will take for referrals, assessments and investigations to be carried out can also provide an estimated discharge date.	Review Linda's plan of care and clinical presentation, as her symptoms have resolved then, once all her assessments are complete, she can be discharged. Keep Linda up to date with progress so that she can begin to plan for discharge.
6. Review the discharge plan each day with the patient and update progress towards discharge date	Review the patient's care plan daily to ensure that it is being met; discuss this with the patient. Take any necessary action to ensure that the care plan is being implemented and update the patient on discharge planning progress.	Discuss Linda's discharge with her each day, ensure that referrals have taken place, discuss with Linda any concerns she has about going home.
7. Involve patients and carers to make informed decisions about care to maximise independence	Involve the patient, and carer, throughout the discharge process. Using ICPs can support planning and delivery of care. If the person has complex discharge planning needs liaise with community services and offer a carer assessment.	Keep Linda up to date with her discharge plans.
8. Plan discharges and transfers to take place over 7 days	This approach promotes timely discharge and spreads the discharge load evenly across the week, avoiding peaks (Friday) and troughs (Monday).	Notify Linda that she may be discharged during the weekend; this might suit Linda better as her son will be available for a couple of days before returning to work on a Monday.

Step	Key points	Application to Linda
9. Use a discharge checklist 24–48 hours pre discharge	Using a checklist allows for a record of all actions taken to be recorded; they can improve communication between the MD and the patient and family or carers. A checklist could include when aspects of care such as medication and transport have been ordered/received.	Complete Linda's discharge checklist paying particular attention to medication. Discuss transport options with her.
10. Make decisions to discharge/ transfer each day	While the overall legal responsibility for a patient's care remains with the senior medical practitioner, nurses can take responsibility for initiating simple discharges. A key factor for this is the patient's 'clinical stability' and their need for 'hospital type' assessment and treatment.	Linda remains clinically stable with her condition improving. She understands her new medication and the need to adapt her diet.

Table 6.4: The DH 10-step framework applied to Linda's discharge planning

Discharge planning is a crucial aspect of patient care; however it is recognised that it does not always happen in a timely and organised manner. Take the time to complete Activity 6.4. This activity will allow you to examine your local discharge policy/protocol and explore some of the reasons why discharge planning is successful or not.

Activity 6.5   *Evidence-based practice and research*

During your next practice learning experience locate your local discharge policy/protocol and associated documentation, for example discharge checklist, and familiarise yourself with it. Then answer the following questions.

1. Is the discharge policy/protocol followed?

If you answered yes to this question then go to question 2; if you answered no then go to question 3.

2. Why is this – are there specific strategies/attitudes in place to ensure it is followed?
3. Why is this – what prevents the discharge policy/protocol being followed?

If you answered question 2 then go to question 4; if you answered question 3 then go to question 5.

(Continued)

(Continued)

4. How could this area of good practice be shared with other clinical areas?
5. What could be done to improve the discharge planning process in this area?

As the answers will be based on your own observations there is no outline answer at the end of this chapter.

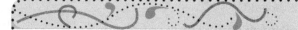

Chapter summary

This chapter has provided you with an overview of complex care in LTCs and how it is managed. It has outlined the important role case management plays in promoting proactive care and in increasing satisfaction in those living with an LTC, and applied this to your clinical practice. ICPs have been explored in relation to the care and management of those with LTCs; using ICPs ensures that an appropriate plan of care is provided. The importance of effective medicines optimisation has been acknowledged and the role of medicines review discussed. Discharge planning has been highlighted with the emphasis being placed on the discharge planning process and the importance of this being a planned and timely event.

Having read this chapter, worked through the activities and accessed the further reading you will have developed your knowledge and skills in relation to how complex care, in LTCs, is managed. By having an understanding of the role and responsibilities of the case manager you can liaise effectively with members of the multidisciplinary team to provide an appropriate level of care. By accessing and using ICPs you can ensure that those living with LTCs receive evidence-based care at the right time, in the right place and by the right person. Recognising the importance of the discharge planning process will enable you to work with those living with an LTC and their carers to address relevant concerns and issues.

Further reading

Cubby, A and Bowler, M (2010) Community matrons and long-term conditions: an inside view. *British Journal of Community Nursing*, 15 (2): 71–6.

Department of Health (2010) *Ready to Go? Planning the Discharge and Transfer of Patients from Hospital and Intermediate Care*. Leeds: Department of Health.
This guide explains the 10 key steps to achieving a safe and timely discharge, and is aimed at both health and social care professionals.

Knight, DA, Thompson, BA, Mathie, E and Dickinson, A (2011) 'Seamless care? Just a list would have helped!' Older people and their carer's experiences of support with medication on discharge from hospital. *Health Expectations*, 16: 277–91.
A qualitative research article exploring older people's, and their carers', experiences of hospital discharge in relation to medicines management.

Useful websites

www.housinglin.org.uk/hospital2home_pack

This website provides useful information to support discharge planning and complements the DH 10-step framework.

www.institute.nhs.uk/building_capability/general/aims.html

The home page for High Impact Actions: The Essential Collection. It contains useful information and examples of case studies.

http://pathways.nice.org.uk

This website provides information on a range of care pathways. They are easy to access and provide an up-to-date evidence-based resource for health and social care professionals

Chapter 7
Palliative care in long term conditions

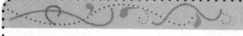

By entry to the register:

13. Uses appropriate and relevant communication skills to deal with difficult and challeng-ing circumstances, for example, responding to emergencies, unexpected occurrences, saying 'no', dealing with complaints, resolving disputes, de-escalating aggression, conveying 'unwelcome news'.

Cluster: Organisational aspects of care

9. People can trust the newly registered graduate nurse to treat them as partners and work with them to make a holistic and systematic assessment of their needs; to develop a personalised plan that is based on mutual understanding and respect for their indi-vidual situation promoting health and wellbeing, minimising risk of harm and promoting their safety at all times.

By entry to the register:

16. Promotes health and wellbeing, self-care and independence by teaching and empower-ing people and carers to make choices in coping with the effects of treatment and the ongoing nature and likely consequences of a condition including death and dying.

Chapter aims

After reading this chapter you will be able to:

- discuss and apply the principles of breaking bad news to the care and management of people living with an LTC;
- explain what palliative care is and its role in the management of LTCs;
- explain strategies to support palliative and end of life care and their relevance to people living with LTCs;
- recognise the importance of holistic assessment for palliative care in the management of LTCs.

Introduction

You matter to us because you are you, and you matter to the last moment of your life. We will do all we can not only to help you die peacefully, but also to live until you die.

(Dame Cicely Saunders, 1994)

As mentioned in Chapter 1, the incidence of LTCs is rising; there are many LTCs where the trajectory of the condition is such that there will come a time when all curative treatment options have been tried. Traditionally this has meant that there was a specific point in a person's journey when their treatment and care moved from curative to palliative. Nowadays it is generally accepted that supportive and palliative care should start at diagnosis of a life-threatening illness, or LTC, and run alongside curative/active treatment. Initially supportive and palliative care may be a small part of the care and management of LTCs and will run alongside health promotion, self-care and symptom management. However, as the person's LTC progresses, and symptom management becomes increasingly difficult as the disease burden increases, supportive and palliative care will play a larger role in their care and management. Whether the emphasis on supportive and palliative care, rather than curative treatment, comes early or late in a person's journey, it is important that they are provided with the knowledge to enable them to make informed decisions about their care and that they are able to discuss their fears and desires with those caring for them.

Talking about death and dying is not something we are comfortable about as it reminds us of our own mortality; however, effectively supporting people receiving palliative care requires you to become involved and empathise with the person and their situation. Utilising the knowledge and skills developed in Chapter 2 will enable you to recognise your own fears as well as those of the people in your care, allowing you to effectively support both individuals living with LTCs and those who care for them.

As the above quote emphasises, palliative care is about focusing on the person and enabling them to carry on 'living' until they die. The point where a person's care becomes more palliative and less curative should not be seen as the end of the journey. Rather it should be viewed as a time when support is provided to enable the person to remain as active and as involved in their life and community for as long as possible and to die a 'good' death. This chapter will help you to develop your knowledge about palliative care and related areas so that you can feel more confident about caring for people during this important time. It will help you to source the relevant skills and information so that you are better equipped to enable people in the end stages of their life to live and die in the place of their choice and in a manner appropriate for them.

Breaking bad news in long term conditions

Chapter 1 introduced you to the concept of physical and psychological 'noise' in your communication with people living with LTCs. The impact of 'noise' was discussed in relation to the delivery of a diagnosis of an LTC and its perception as being 'bad news'. Bad news was described as any news that implies the loss of something that an individual values, such as physical ability, or that is life-changing, affecting an individual's perception of themselves in a negative way. For many people living with an LTC, the fact that their treatment is now being described as 'palliative' rather than 'curative' can be seen as further bad news, and this is compounded by the fact that they are now faced with the realisation that they are entering the final stages of their journey.

Breaking bad news is a complex but necessary part of the care and management of people living with LTCs. As well as breaking the bad news the person delivering the news has to prepare themselves for the emotional reaction of the person and their family. They will have to be prepared to answer questions, such as, 'How long do I have?', 'Is there anything else that can be done?' In addition they will have to provide information about future care and management, and ensure that what they have said has been understood.

Although breaking bad news can be difficult and unpleasant for both the healthcare professional and the person receiving the news, it is important. It helps to maintain trust in the therapeutic relationship, reduces uncertainty ('At least I know what I am dealing with'), prevents the build-up of inappropriate hope ('Is there something I should be doing?'), allows the person and their family time to adjust and allows for open communication between the healthcare professionals, the person and their family (Kaye, 1996). Additionally it should be remembered that most patients want to have information about their prognosis, treatment and possible outcome.

Activity 7.1   *Reflection*

Whether it is breaking bad news or answering awkward questions, many healthcare professionals find this difficult to do. Either on your own or with a group of your peers, reflect back on your clinical experience and identify a situation where you have been asked an awkward question that you did not feel comfortable answering. Now answer the following questions.

- What was it about the situation that made it awkward?
- How did you respond to the person's question?
- Would you do it differently now?

As the answers will be based on your own observations there is no outline answer at the end of this chapter.

Activity 7.1 will have demonstrated to you that there are many reasons why healthcare professionals feel uncomfortable when breaking bad news or answering awkward questions. They are reminded of their own mortality, they are worried about saying the wrong thing or they are unprepared for the reaction of the person. Some questions that may be useful for you to use in a similar situation to the one reflected on in Activity 7.1 are as follows.

- 'What makes you ask me this question?'
- 'What do you already understand about your condition?'
- 'Would it help you to know more about your condition?'
- 'Would you like to have a member of your family with you when you find out more about your condition?'

This approach will enable you to explore the person's concerns without having to give information that you may not feel capable or competent to deliver. Given the complexities of breaking bad news, some approaches have been developed to support and guide the process (Baile et al., 2000; Narayanan et al., 2010).

Approaches to use when breaking bad news in LTCs

Bad news should be delivered in a sensitive manner, allowing the person to feel that they have been listened to and understood. The person, and their carer and family, should leave knowing what the plan for their future care and treatment is. To support healthcare professionals in breaking bad news, specific approaches have been developed. These include Baile et al.'s SPIKES 6-step protocol (2000) and Narayanan et al.'s BREAKS protocol (2010). While both these protocols make the assumption that 'breaking bad news' can be planned for in the setting/background step this is not always the case. As you may know from your clinical practice, and as reflected on in Activity 7.1, patients often ask questions on the spur of the moment. Whether you are able to plan for the conversation or not, what is important is that both these protocols can be used to support sensitive, person-centred communication. Table 7.1 outlines both Baile et al.'s SPIKES 6-step protocol (2000) and Narayanan et al's BREAKS protocol (2010) and applies them to your practice.

SPIKES 6-step protocol (Baile et al., 2000)	BREAKS protocol (Narayanan et al., 2010)	Areas to consider
Setting	Background	Know all the facts before the consultation, including patient's emotional state and support system; ensure privacy and comfort, switch off mobile phones and allow time for the meeting. Check that all the appropriate people are there; remember in some cultures it would be expected that the head of the family be present.
Perception	Rapport	Ask the person what they understand is happening: 'Do you know why we are meeting today?'
		Use open questions to develop a rapport; ask for a narrative of events from the person to determine their perception of the illness: 'Could you tell me . . .' or 'How did it all start?' Allow the person to complete
	Exploring	their narrative before asking questions, listen to what they are saying and identify cues to explore further. Avoid making premature reassurances; explore the patient's (and family's) understanding of their condition and beliefs about their situation.
Invitation		Obtain permission for the person for more information: 'Would you like me to explain a bit more?' Remember that for the person it can be

		frightening asking for more information – how much do they want to know?
Knowledge	Announce	Warn first about sharing bad news: 'I'm afraid this is rather serious' or 'The news is not what we had hoped for'. Be aware of non-verbal communication; adopt an open body position. Denial is a natural coping mechanism: allow the person to control how much information is given. Narrow the information gap by providing information in simple language; check understanding before continuing. Avoid being blunt, giving incomplete information or false hope. The detail may not be remembered but how you gave the information will be.
Emotion	Kindling	People will respond in different ways; allow for expression of feelings. Some may want to get up and move around, others might respond with 'black' humour; allow time for this emotional outlet. Respond with empathy: 'What are your main concerns at the moment?' and address the person's concerns and emotions: 'This must be difficult for you'; explore and validate the person's feelings: 'It is only natural that you feel this way'. For the person, this is the most important part in relation to their satisfaction with the meeting. Be alert to differential listening, when the patient only hears what they want to hear; identify areas to revisit at a later date.
Summary	Summarise	Review the information discussed and provide a summary, written if necessary. Answer questions, and discuss options and plans for future care. Offer availability: some details may not be remembered, further support will be needed and they may need time to talk to family. If the person is on their own, find out if there is someone that they would like to have contacted.

Table 7.1: Areas to consider when using Baile et al.'s SPIKES 6-step protocol (2000) and Narayanan et al.'s BREAKS protocol (2010)

As both the protocols discussed in Table 7.1 identify in the summary/summarise sections, breaking bad news should not be a one-off event. Rather patients, and their carer/families, should be provided with a further opportunity to meet with healthcare staff to discuss their situation and have any concerns and questions answered.

Using a previous experience from your clinical practice when you have witnessed 'bad news' being broken, identify if either Baile et al.'s SPIKES 6-step protocol or Narayanan et al.'s BREAKS was used. If they were used how effective were they? If they were not used, then how would using this protocol have improved the situation?

As the answers will be based on your own observations there is no outline answer at the end of this chapter.

Using the approaches outlined in Table 7.1 should help you to improve the process of breaking bad news, both for the person delivering the bad news and for the person receiving the bad news. When undertaking Activity 7.2 you may have reflected on how the person receiving the bad news reacted to the news.

Breaking bad news to people with a learning disability

It is recognised that certain groups of people require information to be provided in a different format, for example those with cognitive impairment, e.g., learning disability. Tuffrey-Wijne (2012) noted that 'step' based protocols were not appropriate for people with an LD where, for example, it can be difficult to establish a person's level of knowledge. Following research Tuffrey-Wijne (2012) proposed new guidelines that recognise breaking bad news to people with an LD is an ongoing process where knowledge is discussed in blocks and built on over time. Her guidelines incorporate the following areas:

- Understanding – this focuses on the issue of capacity; to do this it is important that you are aware of the legislation around capacity and how it applies to the individual person's situation. It is generally accepted that everyone is assumed to have capacity unless it can be proved otherwise. Having capacity means that a person has the ability to understand information, retain this and use it to make a specific decision. Knowing how much a person understands is important as it will determine when and how bad news is broken.

- People – all people involved in the care of a person with an LD have a role to play in assisting the person to understand what has been said. Using a carer's knowledge of how a person communicates and their life history can support the person breaking the bad news to identify what blocks of information should be given and when. It is also important to take into consideration the views of the carer; however this should not focus on their 'wishes', for example, they may not want the person to be told the bad news. However, everyone who has capacity has the right to be given information, unless they choose otherwise.

- Support – this includes support for the person with an LD and their family and carers; it should be recognised that in some cases formal carers may have been looking after the person for some time and will have developed a close therapeutic relationship with them. Ongoing support for the person with an LD will be needed; therefore it is important that those caring for them are equipped with the knowledge and skills to do this.

Within these guidelines it is recognised that capacity can change and that this should be reviewed at every interaction. However sensitively bad news is broken the reaction of the person, and their family, to the news can be unpredictable. Knowing the person and how they have reacted to previous bad news will help you to support them during this stage.

Reactions to bad news

From your previous clinical, and life, experiences you will be aware that people react to hearing bad news in a variety of ways. Their initial reactions may include denial ('I don't believe this'), numbness ('This can't be happening'), anger ('I knew there was something wrong, if only the tests had been carried out sooner') and grief. A person's reactions depend on the size of the loss and their usual coping mechanisms. How well they have coped with previous 'bad news' and changes in the status of their LTC will be an indicator as to how well they will cope with the news that their treatment is changing from curative to palliative. Many people put on a 'brave face' and, at the time of hearing the news, are able to conduct a rational dialogue, asking for further information and rechecking what has already been said. This is their way of confirming the reality of their situation as psychologically they struggle to come to terms with the news. However, as noted in Table 7.1, it is likely that they will not remember the details of the consultation and the information provided, therefore it is important to review their understanding at a later date. Early reactions to the news such as anger, guilt and sadness may also be present; anger may be expressed towards family and members of the healthcare team. You should remember that the person is not angry with you but at the news that has been delivered. Once the initial reaction to the news has passed, some later reactions and coping mechanisms that people display include:

- fighting spirit – 'I will not let this beat me';
- stoical acceptance – 'this is how it is and I will just have to get on with it';
- denial – 'there is nothing wrong with me';
- resigned helplessness – 'what is the point in doing anything, the damage is already done'.

Perhaps the most definitive work that researched people's responses to bad news is that of Elisabeth Kübler-Ross, who in 1969 completed a study that focused on people's reactions to their own dying and death. During this study she interviewed over 200 people about their thoughts and feelings in relation to their dying and death. The result of this work was the five stages of dying: denial, anger, bargaining, depression and acceptance (Kübler-Ross, 2009). It should be noted that Kübler-Ross emphasised that these were the stages people may go through and that they may not progress through them in a linear manner.

> The stages have evolved since their introduction, and they have been very misunderstood over the past three decades. They were never meant to help tuck messy emotions into neat packages. They are responses to loss that many people have, but there is not a typical response to loss, as there is no typical loss. Our grief is as individual as our lives. Not everyone goes through all of them or in a prescribed order.

(Kübler-Ross, 2005, p. 7)

While Kübler-Ross does provide you with a framework, you should remember that it is not always easy to separate out the emotional (anger) and the cognitive (acceptance) and that these can be interdependent and displayed at the same time. Additionally people may display other emotions such as disbelief and confusion in addition to anger and depression. Over time the stages of dying have been applied to those who are grieving; however, their relevance to grieving has been questioned. Kübler-Ross stated the bargaining stage was a time when the dying person makes a commitment to something, and is rewarded for this, by their death being postponed. It could be argued that for a bereaved person, it is too late for bargaining as the death has already occurred (Calderwood, 2011). To support you in your care of the bereaved there are many available bereavement theories that are more suited for use with those who are bereaved. See also the further reading list at the end of this chapter. At whatever point in the course of a person's illness bad news is broken, what is important is that their ongoing palliative care needs are met. However, for the progression of some LTCs (e.g. COPD, heart failure), it can be difficult to predict and many people will have lived through many exacerbations of their condition. For example, it is estimated that up to 50% of people with heart failure will die suddenly (Wilmot, 2002). It is essential therefore to ensure that the relevant care and management is in place early for these people, allowing for maximum symptom relief and quality of life.

Palliative care

Palliative care is an approach to a person's care that improves the quality of their life, and that of their carer and family, when they are living with advanced and progressive illness. The term 'palliative' is derived from the Latin word 'pallium', which means 'cloak or cover'; in palliative care a person's symptoms are not cured but 'cloaked' or minimised, through effective symptom management. The aim is to promote comfort, without cure, and to achieve a good quality of life: *May you be wrapped in tenderness, you my brother, as if in a cloak* (Qu'ran). Chapter 5 of this book discusses the use of effective care planning in symptom management; the same principles should be applied when managing symptoms in palliative care. Quality of life is improved through the early identification of problems and the accurate assessment and treatment of them. Problems may be physical (e.g. pain), psychological (e.g. fear), social (e.g. stigma) and spiritual (e.g. loss of meaning). WHO (2002, p. 84) states that palliative care:

- provides relief from pain and other distressing symptoms;
- affirms life and regards dying as a natural process;
- intends neither to hasten nor postpone death;
- integrates the psychosocial and spiritual aspects of patient care;
- offers a support system to help patients live as actively as possible until death;
- offers a support system to help the family cope during the patient's illness and in their own bereavement;
- uses a team approach to address the needs of patients and their families, including bereavement counselling, if indicated;

- will enhance quality of life, and may also positively influence the course of illness;

- is applicable early in the course of illness, in conjunction with other therapies that are intended to prolong life, such as chemotherapy or radiation therapy, and includes those investigations needed to better understand and manage distressing clinical complications.

Given that the disease progression of different LTCs varies – some people experience a sudden decline, others experience both a gradual decline and acute episodes and some have a steady yet progressive decline – it is important to view palliative care as part of the continuum of care people living with LTCs receive. As a person's LTC progresses and their symptoms increase, treatment that is aimed at modifying the LTC decreases, and at this point palliative care increases, providing support for the person and their carer and family before, during and after the person's death (see Figure 7.1).

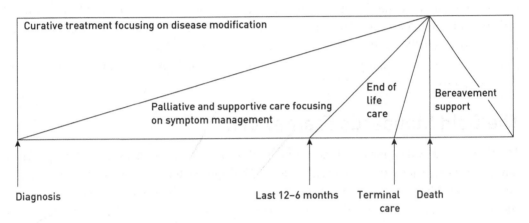

Figure 7.1: The need for care before, during and after a person's death

Activity 7.3 *Reflection*

Either on your own, or with a colleague, reflect on the care and management of a person living with an LTC and write down/discuss whether the diagram in Figure 7.1 represents how palliative care was used as part of the person's care and management, taking into consideration the following:

- Was this representation of palliative care used; if so how?
- If it was not used, why was this and what difference might it have made to the person's care and management?

As the answers will be based on your own observations there is no outline answer at the end of this chapter.

While there is a specific chapter in this book relating to palliative and end of life care, hopefully Activity 7.3 will have allowed you to see that palliative and end of life care are integral parts of a person's care and management. This approach means that palliative care is not delivered in a specific care setting; it can be delivered in a number of settings, e.g. a person's own home, nursing home or a hospice. Neither is it provided by one specific group of healthcare professionals: it is provided by many, including Macmillan nurses, district nurses, GPs and healthcare professionals working in secondary and tertiary care.

Strategies to support palliative and end of life care for people with LTCs

To promote the delivery of person-centred and timely palliative care there are a range of recognised strategies available that you can use. These strategies support both the strategic care and management, how a clinical team might organise the care and management of this group of patients and face to face care. These include: the Gold Standards Framework (GSF), preferred priorities of care (PPC) and advance care planning (ACP). The timing of conversations around palliative care are crucial; a precondition for this is how much the person understands about their prognosis (Munday et al., 2009).

The Gold Standards Framework

The GSF is a UK-wide approach that can be used to support you to deliver effective palliative care in a primary care setting. You can apply the GSF approach to any person, in any setting; it focuses on enabling people to live well in the last years, months or days of their life (Thomas, 2003). The main focus of the GSF is to enable you, as part of a primary healthcare team, to work collaboratively to maximise a person's continuity of care, introduce ACP, promote symptom control and provide ongoing support. Through the use of GP practice based palliative care registers, linked in to the Quality Outcome Framework (see Chapter 1), those receiving palliative care are easily identified to all members of the practice team, improving communication and the care received. The GSF will be discussed further in this chapter in the section on delivering holistic palliative care; the web link for the GSF website can be found in the useful websites section at the end of this chapter.

Preferred priorities for care

A systematic review on adult preferences for place of care at end of life or place of death carried out in 2013 (Gomes et al., 2013) identified that between 52–92% of people not diagnosed with a 'life-threatening illness' would prefer to die at home. It could be said that asking this question to people who are not faced with the reality that they will die may not provide a true reflection of what actually occurs. This could be especially true if the lead up to a person's death is sudden or particularly challenging to manage. However a narrative appraisal of people's preferences in relation to dying at home by Higginson et al. (2013) found that for the majority of people approaching the end of their life home remains their preferred place of care and that this preference remains stable as their condition deteriorates. Currently, however, the majority of people do not die in their own home; 54% of people die in hospital, meaning that approximately

60–70% of people do not die in their preferred place (Royal College of General Practitioners, 2013). To address this challenge advance care planning was introduced, with the preferred priorities for care process being part of this.

Completing a PPC is a voluntary process. The completed document is kept by the person receiving palliative care, and the information on the PPC is shared with those planning and delivering their care. It documents aspects of their future care that is important to them, such as 'Where would you like to be cared for in the future?' and 'What are your priorities for your future care?' and focuses on the person's beliefs and values. You can then use this information to ensure that the care you deliver takes into account what is important to that person. Relevant information from the PCC can also be used in future care planning. This is particularly useful should a person receiving palliative care no longer be able to make decisions themselves, for example a person with dementia or a degenerative neurological condition. It should not be used to record information relating to refusal of medical treatment, as the PPC is not a legally binding document. However it is recognised under the Mental Capacity Act (2005), if a person has already completed a PCC, and no longer has capacity to make decisions, the information recorded in their PCC should be taken into account. You should endeavour to ensure that a person keeps their PCC up to date as their wishes and views may change over time (Cancer Research UK, 2014). For those living with dementia or a degenerative neurological condition, and who lack mental capacity, it may be necessary to discuss having a lasting power of attorney (LPA)/power of attorney (PoA). An LPA/PoA is a document that allows people living with LTCs to choose someone to make decisions on their behalf when they lack the mental capacity to do so themselves. Within the UK there may be slight variations in law as it relates to LPA/PoA and mental capacity, therefore you will need to familiarise yourself with the law as it relates to mental capacity and LPA/PoA in the country where you work.

Advance care planning (ACP)

ACP is a voluntary process that allows for an open and structured discussion between the person receiving palliative care and those caring for them, including their family and carer. While these might have occurred informally ACP allows for the person's preferences to be recorded and communicated between members of the health and social care team. ACP differs from traditional care planning, which addresses current areas of need, such as reduced nutritional intake and how they are to be managed. ACP addresses a person's anticipated deterioration and what their preferences for treatment would be; this is especially relevant should the person's ability to communicate reduce or their capacity to make decisions deteriorate (GSF, 2015). As such ACP is recognised within the Mental Capacity Act (2005); the purpose of the discussion is to discuss and document the following (GMC, 2013):

- the person's wishes and concerns;
- the person's values and beliefs;
- the family members, and others close to the person or LPA/PoA that the person would like involved in decisions about their treatment;
- interventions that might be considered in an emergency, such as admission to hospital and cardiopulmonary resuscitation, when it may be helpful for a decision to be made in advance;

- the person's preferred place of care;
- the person's need for religious, spiritual or other personal support.

It is important that any discussions you have are documented, reviewed regularly and communicated to appropriate people, including the person's carer and family, if required. Within the ACP framework there are two ways in which a person can state their preferences regarding their future care and management; these are (1) a statement of wishes and preferences; and (2) an advance decision to refuse treatment. Before discussing either of these options with a person in your care it is essential that you have an understanding of mental capacity and its relevance to ACP. Within the UK there may be slight variations in law as it relates to ACP and mental capacity, therefore you will need to familiarise yourself with the law as it relates to mental capacity and ACP in the country where you work.

Statement of wishes and preferences

A statement of wishes and preferences allows the person living with an LTC, who is in the palliative stages of their illness, to either write down or verbally express, and have documented, their wishes and preferences in relation to future treatment. This may take the form of explaining their feelings, beliefs and values that influence how they make decisions. It may also include areas of a person's care such as where they would like to be cared for, and what types of treatment they are prepared to have. While this is not a legally binding document, it does have legal standing as part of the Mental Capacity Act (MCA, 2005) and should be taken into account when deciding on a person's future treatment options.

Advance decision to refuse treatment

Some people living with LTCs may have strong feelings about specific treatments they would not want to have. In order to have this recognised it is necessary for an advance decision to refuse treatment (an Advance Directive) to be made. An advance decision to refuse treatment is a legally binding document and is part of the MCA (2005) and should only be made under the guidance of a healthcare professional who understands the process. It only applies if the person making the decision is over the age of 18 and has the mental capacity to make the necessary decision and will only come into effect if the person loses their capacity to make decisions about their treatment. An advance decision to refuse treatment allows the person to specifically express, and have documented, the type of medical treatment they wish to refuse, e.g. being treated with antibiotics for a chest infection. It must relate to specific treatments and circumstances and will only come into effect at these times (The National Council for Palliative Care (NCPC), 2008).

ACP is a voluntary process that should be initiated by the person receiving the care. It should be handled sensitively and by a healthcare professional who has a clear understanding of the person's clinical condition, treatments options and side effects and the legal and ethical issues involved. If you are uncertain about any of these, or lack the required knowledge, then ask a colleague who does to lead the discussions. To enable open and honest communication during palliative and end of life care the importance of developing a therapeutic relationship cannot be underestimated. Whether it is a conversation about PCC or ACP, discussions around palliative care should be carried out by those who have a rapport with the person and their family. The aspects of the EoLC strategy outlined above are there to support you in your delivery of appropriate and effective palliative care to people living with an LTC. Regardless of whether the person you are caring for has made explicit their preferences for care, ensuring that they are assessed correctly and that the care delivered meets their needs is your priority.

Activity 7.4   *Teamwork*

Delivering holistic palliative care requires a multidisciplinary approach. Write down a list of all the people you think are involved in delivering palliative care. Reading Table 7.2 might provide you with some prompts.

An outline answer to this activity is given at the end of the chapter.

As your answer to Activity 7.4 will have identified, a whole range of people are involved in delivering palliative care. Some of these may be specialist practitioners, however many of them will be generalists working in primary or secondary care.

Holistic palliative care in long term conditions

Palliative care is delivered by a variety of healthcare professionals in a variety of settings. Palliative care can be provided by both generalist and specialist healthcare professionals. Generalists should be able to provide the day-to-day care for people requiring palliative care, their carer and family through effective assessment, management and appropriate referral to specialist services. Specialists, such as palliative care consultants and clinical nurse specialists, are healthcare professionals with a high level of knowledge and skill in the field of palliative care who are responsible for directing a plan of care that allows for the integration of available resources and services. This may include providing care and management in the person's home or in a local hospice, and bereavement support.

Assessing for holistic palliative care

To enable both generalists and specialists to provide coordinated care to the person requiring palliative care and their family, it is important to fully assess the person and their needs. The GSF recommends the use of the PEPSICOLA approach while the End of Life Care Programme (NHS Improving Quality, 2010) recommends the use of a holistic common assessment. Both these frameworks will enable you to undertake a person-centred holistic assessment. Table 7.2 provides an overview of the PEPSICOLA approach and the holistic common assessment with prompts for you to consider.

PEPSICOLA	Holistic common assessment	Prompts to consider
P – physical	Physical wellbeing: the aim is to identify all potential needs, so a review of all aspects of physical health is required.	Assess symptoms and overall management plan, review medication and stop non-essential treatment. Identify the person's priorities: is there a specific concern, what effect is this having on their ADLs, discuss options and explore any fears.
E – emotional	Psychological wellbeing: the recognition of psychological needs, not specialist assessment.	Consider what the person knows about their condition, how they and their family are coping and what signifies deterioration for that person. What impact is this having on the person and their family, what have they done to manage their situation, e.g., relaxation; what else could be done?
P – personal	Spiritual wellbeing: it is important to lead in to this assessment; if you do not feel comfortable undertaking this assessment then ask another member of the team.	Recognise cultural background, language, sexuality, spirituality and religious needs, and find out their beliefs and faith. Has their situation affected these, identify any requirements for spiritual support, does the person have any life goals they would like to achieve?
S – social support	Social and occupational wellbeing: home and community, work and finance, family and close relations and social and recreational.	Carry out a DS1500 assessment and carer assessment if not already completed; where is the person's PCC? Identify what support the person is receiving and does this need reviewing?
I – information and communication		Communication between the person and the healthcare team and vice versa; how will the healthcare team communicate with each other? Is the person aware of the plans and do they understand them?
C – control and autonomy		Consider mental capacity and discuss treatment options, including, if required, PCC and ACP. Is there any conflict between the person and their family/carer?
O – out-of-hours		Does the person know who to contact during out-of-hours, and what carer support is available? Consider medication for use out-of-hours.

| L – late | | Terminal care (last 2 days): is the person comfortable, are they and their family aware of the situation, has all non-essential medication/treatment been stopped? |
| A – after | | Planning for bereavement, information and support for family and carer, inform other members of the healthcare team. |

Table 7.2: Areas to consider when completing an assessment using either PEPSICOLA (Thomas, 2003) or the holistic common assessment (NHS Improving Quality, 2010)

Case study: Andrew

Despite trying to improve both his levels of exercise and his nutritional intake, Andrew's condition has continued to deteriorate. He has continued to have recurrent chest infections that have reduced his appetite further, increased his level of dyspnoea and drastically reduced his exercise tolerance. Since his last chest infection he has required **long term oxygen therapy** *(LTOT) at home due to reduced oxygen saturation levels. David (Andrew's community matron) has graded his dyspnoea at 4 on the Medical Research Council dyspnoea scale. This indicates that Andrew has to stop for breath after walking about 100 metres or after a few minutes on level ground. His most recent* **spirometry** *result stated that his FEV1 (forced expired volume) was 30%, indicating end-stage COPD. Both Andrew's GP and David are concerned about his deteriorating condition and have asked each other the 'surprise' question: 'Would you be surprised if this person were to die in the next 6–12 months?' They both answered no to this question (RCGP, 2008).*

With the consent of his GP, David has discussed the results of Andrew's spirometry with him, and what this means for his future care with the emphasis being on palliative care. Andrew has said he would like to stay in his flat for as long as possible. However, he is now requiring homecare assistance in the morning and evening to assist him with his personal hygiene. He has meals on wheels five days of the week and a neighbour in the sheltered housing cooks a meal for him at the weekend. He is finding the change in his situation rather lonely as he is not able to get out and about. He has begun to talk about his wife Elizabeth recently.

Activity 7.5   *Critical thinking*

Drawing upon the above information and the information in Chapter 6, use the PEPSICOLA/holistic common assessment framework to assess Andrew's needs in relation to his palliative care.

A brief outline answer is given at the end of this chapter.

Having used the PEPSICOLA/holistic common assessment framework to assess Andrew's needs (Activity 7.5), and using the nursing process, you are now able to plan and implement an appropriate plan of care that will address his ongoing healthcare needs. Whatever a person's palliative care needs are, what is essential is that through effective communication and collaboration the person and their family receive the best care, by the most appropriate person in the place of their choice.

Delivering holistic palliative care

The GSF incorporates seven standards of care that relate to the effective delivery of holistic palliative care for people living with an LTC. Emphasis is placed on both direct care and management and the management and coordination of the healthcare professionals delivering the care (Thomas, 2003). Table 7.3 outlines these standards and their aims.

GSF standards of care	Aim and areas to consider
Communication	The aim of this standard is to improve *how* information is communicated (written, verbal and electronic) and *who* is involved in any communication (person receiving palliative care, out-of-hours, family, etc.). A supportive care register allows a GP practice to record, monitor and review the care received by people in the last 6–12 months of their life. Through the use of monthly meetings proactive care and management can be planned, with ACP being incorporated if required.
Coordination	The aim of this standard is to ensure that the care delivered to people requiring palliative care is well organised and coordinated with communication being maintained. Each PHCT should have a nominated palliative care coordinator, e.g., practice nurse, district nurse. The palliative care coordinator is responsible for maintaining relevant paperwork, including the supportive care register, arranging the monthly meetings and ensuring appropriate tools such as PEPSICOLA are used.
Control of symptoms	The aim of this standard is to promote effective symptom management through the use of appropriate assessment such as PEPSICOLA. Each person receiving palliative care is assured of having a holistic assessment with the results being discussed and an appropriate person-centred plan of care being devised.
Continuity	The aim of this standard is to ensure continuity of care during out-of-hours, ensuring that the person receiving palliative care is supported during out-of-hours. Using the protocol devised by Calderdale and Kirklees Health Authority (Thomas, 2003) will promote continuity of care. It addresses four key areas:

	• communication – between GP/district nurse and out-of-hours service; • carer support – does the carer know what to do in a crisis, is a night sitter required? • medical support – any anticipated management documented in handover form; • drugs/equipment – leave any anticipated medication in person's home.
Continued learning	The aim of this standard is to promote reflective learning or 'learning as you go' to further develop the care given to people receiving palliative care. Through the use of practice-based teaching, significant event analysis and other learning opportunities, the professional development of those caring for people requiring palliative care is enhanced. Learning should focus on all areas of palliative care: strategic (planning of resources/ coordination of services), clinical (treatment/management options) and personal (communication skills).
Carer support	The aim of this standard is to improve carer support: carers are key in enabling people receiving palliative care to remain in their own home. Through the provision of emotional and practical support carers are empowered to play as active a part as they would like to. Carer support does not stop when the person dies: bereavement support should be offered.
Care of the dying (terminal phase)	The aim of this standard is to promote suitable care in the last days of a person's life. Using such tools as the Liverpool Care Pathway for the Dying Patient will ensure that non-essential treatment is stopped, the person's symptoms are controlled and psychological and religious/spiritual support is available.

Table 7.3: The 7Cs of the GSF (based on the work of Thomas, 2003)

Chapter summary

This chapter has provided you with an overview of breaking bad news, palliative care and the EoLC strategy. These important areas are all key aspects of the care and management of people living with an LTC. It has outlined some approaches that can be used when breaking bad news and applied these to your clinical practice. Palliative care and the EoLC strategy have been outlined in relation to providing appropriate care for people living with

(Continued)

(Continued) •

an LTC. Finally the importance of undertaking a holistic assessment has been discussed and applied to your clinical practice.

Having read through this chapter and undertaken the activities, you will have developed your knowledge and skills in relation to the principles of breaking bad news, palliative care, the EoLC strategy and how to assess a person's holistic palliative care needs. How you use the information in this chapter will depend on where you are working and your current roles and responsibilities. However, as a nurse, you can ensure that planning for palliative care becomes part of your overall care and management of people living with an LTC. By having an increased awareness of some of the approaches that can be used when breaking bad news you will be better able to answer awkward questions and support those in your care. Increasing your knowledge of palliative care and the EoLC strategy will allow you to provide appropriate and relevant information to both the person living with an LTC and their carer, allowing them to make informed choices. Using frameworks such as PEPSICOLA will promote the delivery of person-centred holistic care that meets the ongoing needs of the person, their carer and family.

Activities: brief outline answers

Activity 7.4 Teamwork (page 147)

You might have listed the following people as being part of the multidisciplinary team: clinical nurse specialist, district nurse, general practitioner, speech and language therapist, palliative care consultant, occupational therapist, physiotherapist, chaplain, counsellor, pharmacist, dietician, family support worker, the patient, their family and carer, complementary therapist, school nurse, community psychiatric nurse and practice nurse.

Activity 7.5 Critical thinking (page 149)

P – physical	Review of Andrew's medication, use of bronchodilators and inhaled corticosteroids. Ongoing LTOT assessment and review: ensure Andrew is aware of the health and safety issues. Comprehensive assessment regarding other possible symptoms, e.g. pain, nutritional intake.
E – emotional	Having spoken to his community matron, Andrew is aware that his condition has deteriorated. He is concerned about being on his own as he is no longer able to get out and about as much as he could. Andrew has started talking about his wife Elizabeth recently; this may mean he is beginning to think about his own death. It is essential that Andrew knows who and how to contact people should his condition deteriorate. If he does not have one then a pendant alarm would be appropriate.
P – personal	We don't know a lot about Andrew's personal beliefs; this is the time to begin to discuss these with him. It may be useful to find out what kind of funeral service he arranged for Elizabeth.

S – social support	Is Andrew claiming all the available benefits; has a DS1500 been completed? Social isolation is a potential problem; Andrew enjoys company but may become increasingly isolated due to his dyspnoea. Does he have all the necessary aids at home to promote his independence? Andrew has indicated that he would like to stay in his flat for as long as possible; how to manage this and alternatives may have to be discussed.
I – information and communication	Does Andrew hold a copy of his case notes; are they accessible to all relevant members of the PHCT? Andrew has a community matron; does he know how to contact her? Andrew is aware that his condition is deteriorating, and it may be appropriate to discuss issues such as his will with him.
C – control and autonomy	We do not know what Andrew's thoughts are on his future care apart from the fact that he would like to stay in his flat for as long as possible. It is necessary to discuss preferred place of care and advance directives with him to ensure that his wishes are met.
O – out-of-hours	Communication between the community matron, GP and OOH service should ensure that all know what to do in the case of a deterioration in Andrew's condition. Andrew should know who and how to contact the out-of-hours service.
L – late	Not yet applicable – though through effective communication and working in partnership with Andrew when the time comes, end of life issues should be able to be discussed to ensure appropriate care.
A – after	This may not be discussed, though allowing Andrew time to talk about Elizabeth and her death may enable to talk to Andrew about his own funeral.

Further reading

Buglass, E (2010) Grief and bereavement theories. *Nursing Standard*, 24 (41): 44–7.

Nicol, J and Nyatanga, B (2014) *Palliative and End of Life Care in Nursing*. London: Sage Publishing.
This book covers a range of topics relating to palliative and end of life care and provides practical advice and support to enhance the knowledge and skills of people caring for people when they are receiving palliative and end of life care.

Warnock, C (2014) Breaking bad news: issues relating to nursing practice. *Nursing Standard*, 28 (45): 51–8.

Useful websites

www.breakingbadnews.org
This website contains useful information about how to break bad news to people with a learning disability.

www.dyingmatters.org
This is the website for Dying Matters aimed at promoting public awareness of dying, death and bereavement. It has a range of useful information for health professionals and the public.

www.goldstandardsframework.org.uk

This is a UK-wide framework aimed at enabling generalists to maximise the care they deliver to people nearing the end of their life. This website provides information regarding all aspects of the GSF, including how to use it in a variety of settings, e.g. continuing care, secondary care, available research and the GSF toolkit.

www.ncpc.org.uk

The National Council for Palliative Care (NCPC) is an umbrella organisation for all those involved in providing, commissioning and using palliative care services in England, Wales and Northern Ireland. Its aim is to promote palliative care for all who need it. This site contains useful information on all aspects of palliative care, including publications.

www.palliativecarescotland.org.uk

This organisation has the same remit as the NCPC but in Scotland; it supports and contributes to the strategic direction of palliative care in Scotland. This site contains information on all aspects of their work, including publications.

www.togetherforshortlives.org.uk

This is the website for the charity Together for Short Lives, which aims to provide information and support for all people caring for children with life-threatening and life-limiting conditions.

Glossary

Atonic: lacking in normal muscle tone.

Autonomy: when a person is able to make decisions about, and take responsibility for, their own situation.

Bullae: a large blister or vesicle.

Clonic: an abnormal neuromuscular activity resulting in alternating muscle relaxation and contraction, for example, tonic–clonic epileptic seizure.

Comorbidity: the presence of one or more diseases and the effect of these diseases on the person.

Concordance: agreement to participate in something, for example, concordance with medication regime, i.e., a person agreeing with the prescriber to take their prescribed medication as directed.

Continuous ambulatory peritoneal dialysis (CAPD): renal dialysis that takes place inside the person's body using their peritoneum as the dialysis membrane. This form of dialysis is done at home, usually four times a day, and takes approximately 30 minutes each time.

Determinants of health: the factors that affect a person's health and include the person's social and economic environment, the person's physical environment and the person's individual characteristics and behaviour.

Distal: situated away from the point of origin or attachment.

Enabling: assisting a person to become able to do something, to make something possible.

Epidemiology: the study of the occurrence, transmission and control of infectious diseases, for example, tuberculosis.

Ethos: the fundamental character or spirit that defines a belief, person, group or community.

Gleason score: a grading system used to help anticipate the prognosis of prostate cancer, using samples of tissue taken during a biopsy.

Hyperplasia: an abnormal increase in cell number.

Hypertrophy: an abnormal increase in the cell size.

Long term oxygen therapy (LTOT): oxygen therapy that is usually delivered for a minimum of 15 hours per day, including overnight. Once this is started it is likely that a person will be on this for the rest of their life.

Multimorbidity: the presence of several diseases in the same person at the same time, and the combined effect of these diseases on the person.

Non-blanching erythema: tissue redness that does not turn white when pressure is applied with a finger.

Orthopnea: difficulty in breathing when lying down; it is usually relieved when the person sits or stands up.

Philosophy: the rationale investigation of the truths and principles of reality, knowledge and ethics.

Polyneuropathy: a disorder which affects peripheral nerves which can result in a person experiencing reduced sensation, for example, reduced ability to detect heat.

Polypharmacy: multiple prescriptions, involving different drugs for a number of different conditions.

Primary care: care delivered in or close to a person's home, for example, general practitioner practices, NHS walk in centres and pharmacists.

Prizing: demonstrating that you value and respect someone.

PSA testing: a test which screens for prostate cancer by measuring the level of prostate-specific antigen (PSA) in a man's blood. The normal level of PSA is 4 nanograms (ng)/millilitre of blood, however changes in the level between tests may be a more accurate marker.

Public health: the area of health concerned with the promotion of health and the reduction of health inequalities in the population. It includes the physical, social, mental and economic health of the population.

Respite care: short term temporary care that is arranged to provide a break for those caring for people living with an LTC, for example, residential respite (where nursing or residential care is provided) or domiciliary respite (care is provided in the person's own home).

Secondary care: medical services and hospital care, including elective and emergency care. Access is often via a referral from primary care.

Self-efficacy: a person's belief that they can make a change to their current situation.

Spirometry: a test that determines the breathing capacity of the lungs. It measures both the forced vital capacity (the volume of air expired until a person feels their lungs are empty) and the forced expired volume (the volume of air expired in the first second of expiration).

Status asthmaticus: repeated asthma attacks, without relief, that do not respond to treatment.

Syndrome: disease that has a distinct pattern of signs and symptoms, for example, dementia, Down's syndrome.

Tertiary care: specialised care and treatment that is usually provided in specialist centres.

Tonic: an increase in tone in a person's muscles, for example, contraction or convulsion.

Transient: a condition that is temporary and usually lasts only a short time, for example, a transient ischaemic attack.

References

Achterberg, WP, Pieper, MJC, van Dalen-Kok, AH, de Waal, MWM, Husebo, BS, Lautenbacher, S, Kunz, M, Scherder, EJA and Corbett, A (2013) Pain management in people with dementia. *Clinical Interventions in Aging*, 13 (8): 1471–87.

Adler, R, Rosenfeld, L and Towne, N (1989) *Interplay: The Process of Interpersonal Communication*. Orlando, FL: Rinehart and Winston.

Age UK (2014) *Integrated Care Services: Bringing Together Leaders to Transform Services and Outcomes for People Living with Long-Term Conditions*. [Online] Available from: www.ageuk.org.uk/Documents/EN-GB/For-professionals/Care/Integrated%20Care/Integrated_Services_Report.pdf?epslanguage=en-GB?dtrk=true [Accessed: 23/04/15].

Age UK (2015) *Integrated Care Programme: Our Pathway*. [Online] Available from: www.ageuk.org.uk/professional-resources-home/services-and-practice/integrated-care/pathway [Accessed: 16/05/15].

Allen, D, Channon, S, Lowes, L, Atwell, C and Lane, C (2011) Behind the scenes: the changing role of parents in the transition from child to adult diabetes service. *Diabetic Medicine*, 28 (8): 994–1000.

Alzheimer's Society (2009) *Counting the Cost: Caring for People with Dementia in Hospital Wards*. London: Alzheimer's Society.

Bach, S and Grant, A (2015) *Communication and Interpersonal Skills in Nursing*, 3rd edn. London: Sage/Learning Matters.

Baile, WF, Buckman, R, Lenzi, R, Glober, G, Beale, EA and Kudelka, AP (2000) SPIKES – A six-step protocol for delivering bad news: application to the patient with cancer. *The Oncologist*, 5: 302–11.

Barker, P (2001) The tidal model: the lived-experience in person-centred mental health nursing care. *Nursing Philosophy*, 2: 213–23.

Barrett, D, Wilson, B and Woolands, A (2009) *Care Planning: A Guide for Nurses*. Harlow: Pearson Education.

Bee, PE, Barnes, P and Luker, KA (2008) A systematic review of informal caregivers' needs in providing home-based end-of-life care to people with cancer. *Journal of Clinical Nursing*, 18: 1379–93.

Bentley, A (2014) Case management and long-term conditions: the evolution of community matrons. *British Journal of Community Nursing*, 19 (7): 340–5.

Blunt, I (2013) *Focus on Preventable Admissions: Trends in Emergency Admissions for Ambulatory Care Sensitive Conditions, 2001 to 2013*. London: Health Foundation and Nuffield Trust.

British Geriatric Society (2014) *Fit for Frailty: Consensus Best Practice Guidance for the Care of Older People Living with Frailty in Community and Outpatient Settings*. London: British Geriatric Society.

Brodaty, H (2009) Family caregivers of people with dementia. *Dialogues in Clinical Neuroscience*, 11 (2): 217–28.

Brooker, D and Duce, L (2000) Wellbeing and activity in dementia: a comparison group reminiscence therapy, structured goal-directed group activity and unstructured time. *Age and Mental Health*, 4 (4): 354–8.

Calderwood, K (2011) Adapting the transtheoretical model of change to the bereavement process. *Social Work*, 56 (2): 107–18.

Canadian Institute for Advanced Research (2002) Health Canada, Population and Public Health Branch AB/NWT. In: O'Hara, P (2005) *Discussion Paper: Creating Social and Health Equality – Adopting an Alberta Social Determinants of Health Framework*. Edmonton Social Planning Council. 5.

References

Cancer Research UK (2010) *Prostate Cancer Risks and Causes.* [Online] Available from: www.cancerhelp.org.uk/type/prostate-cancer/about/prostate-cancer-risks-and-causes [Accessed: 10/05/15].

Cancer Research UK (2014) *What Is the Preferred Priorities of Care (PCC) Document?* [Online] Available from: www.cancerresearchuk.org/about-cancer/cancers-in-general/cancer-questions/preferred-priorities-for-care [Accessed: 20/05/15].

Care Quality Commission (2014) *From the Pond in to the Sea: Children's Transition to Adult Health Services.* Gallowgate: Care Quality Commission.

Carers UK (2014a) *Facts about Carers.* [Online] Available from: file:///C:/Users/Jane/Downloads/facts-about-carers–2014.pdf [Accessed: 20/05/15].

Carers UK (2014b) *Carers Manifesto.* London: Carers UK.

Carmichael, F and Hulme, C (2008) Are the needs of carers being met? *Journal of Community Nursing,* 22 (8/9): 4–12.

Carrier, J (2009) *Managing Long-Term Conditions and Chronic Illness in Primary Care: A Guide to Good Practice.* Abingdon: Routledge.

Charon, R and Wyer, P (2008) The art of medicine: narrative evidence-based medicine. *Lancet,* 371: 296–7.

Chen, X, Mao, G and Leng, SX (2014) Frailty syndrome: an overview. *Clinical Interventions in Aging,* 9: 433–41.

Cherniss, C (1998) *Emotional Intelligence: What It Is and Why It Matters.* [Online] Available from: www.eiconsortium.org/pdf/what_is_emotional_intelligence.pdf [Accessed: 07/06/15].

Chilton, S, Melling, K, Drew, D and Clarridge, A (2004) *Nursing in the Community: An Essential Guide to Practice.* London: Hodder Arnold.

Chronic Pain Policy Coalition (2011) *Putting Pain on the Agenda: The Report of the First English Pain Summit.* London: Chronic Pain Policy Coalition.

Clark, D (2002) Between hope and acceptance: the medicalization of dying. *British Medical Journal,* 324 (7342): 905–7.

Clegg, A, Young, J, Iliffe, S, Rikkert, MO and Rockwood, K (2013) Frailty in elderly people. *Lancet,* 381 (868): 752–62.

Clinical Knowledge Summaries (2010a) *HIV Infection and AIDS.* [Online] Available from: http://cks.nice.org.uk/hiv-infection-and-aids#!topicsummary [Accessed: 07/06/15].

Clinical Knowledge Summaries (2010b) *Chronic Obstructive Pulmonary Disease.* [Online] Available from: http://cks.nice.org.uk/chronic-obstructive-pulmonary-disease#!topicsummary [Accessed: 07/06/15].

Clinical Knowledge Summaries (2013) *Asthma.* [Online] Available from: http://cks.nice.org.uk/asthma#!topicsummary [Accessed: 07/06/15].

Clinical Knowledge Summaries (2014a) *Heart Failure: Chronic.* [Online] Available from: http://cks.nice.org.uk/heart-failure-chronic#!backgroundsub:3 [Accessed: 07/06/15].

Clinical Knowledge Summaries (2014b) *Epilepsy: Summary.* [Online] Available from: http://cks.nice.org.uk/epilepsy#!topicsummary [Accessed: 07/06/15].

Clinical Knowledge Summaries (2014c) *Diabetes: Type 1.* [Online] Available from: http://cks.nice.org.uk/diabetes-type–1#!diagnosissub [Accessed: 07/06/15].

Clinical Knowledge Summaries (2014d) *CVD Risk Assessment and Management.* [Online] Available from: http://cks.nice.org.uk/cvd-risk-assessment-and-management#!topicsummary [Accessed: 07/06/15].

Clinical Knowledge Summaries (2015a) *Dementia: Summary.* [Online] Available from: http://cks.nice.org.uk/dementia#!topicsummary [Accessed: 07/06/15].

Clinical Knowledge Summaries (2015b) *Diabetes: Type 2.* [Online] Available from: http://cks.nice.org.uk/diabetes-type–2#!topicsummary [Accessed: 07/06/2015].

ContinYou (2010) *Skilled for Health.* [Online] Available from: www.continyou.org.uk/health_and_well_being/skilled_health [Accessed: 07/06/2015].

Cook, JB (1984) Reminiscing: how can it help confused nursing home residents? *Journal of Contemporary Social Work,* 65: 90–3.

Corben, S and Rosen, R (2005) *Self-Management for Long-Term Conditions: Patient's Perspectives on the Way Ahead.* London: King's Fund.

Coulter, A, Roberts, S and Dixon, A (2013) *Delivering Better Services for People with Long-Term Conditions: Building the House of Care.* [Online] Available from: www.kingsfund.org.uk/sites/files/kf/field/field_publication_file/delivering-better-services-for-people-with-long-term-conditions.pdf [Accessed: 07/06/15].

Dalhgren, G and Whitehead, M (2007) *European Strategies for Tackling Social Inequalities in Health: Levelling Up, Part 2.* Copenhagen: World Health Organization.

Dart, AM (2011) *Motivational Interviewing in Nursing Practice: Empowering the Patient.* London: Jones and Bartlet.

De Silva, D (2011) *Helping People Help Themselves: A Review of the Evidence Considering Whether It Is Worthwhile to Support Self-Management.* London: The Health Foundation.

Department of Health (2005) *Supporting People with Long Term Conditions: An NHS and Social Care Model to Support Local Innovation and Integration.* London: Department of Health.

Department of Health (2006) *Transition: Getting It Right for Young People. Improving the Transition of Young People with Long Term Conditions from Children's to Adult Health Services.* London: Department of Health.

Department of Health (2008a) *High Quality Care for All: NHS Next Stage Review Final Report.* London: The Stationary Office.

Department of Health (2008b) *Raising the Profile of Long Term Conditions Care: A Compendium of Information.* London: Department of Health.

Department of Health (2008c) *Transition: Moving on Well.* 8651. London: Department of Health.

Department of Health (2009) *Living Well with Dementia: A National Dementia Strategy.* London: Department of Health.

Department of Health (2010) *Ready to Go? Planning the Discharge and the Transfer of Patients from Hospital and Intermediate Care.* Leeds: Department of Health.

Department of Health (2012) *Long Term Conditions Compendium of Information,* 3rd edn. London: Department of Health.

Department of Health and NHS Commissioning Board (2012) *Compassion in Practice.* London: Department of Health.

Department of Health, Social Services and Public Safety (2012) *Living With Long Term Conditions: A Policy Framework.* [Online] Available from: www.dhsspsni.gov.uk/living-longterm-conditions.pdf [Accessed: 07/06/15].

DiClemente, CC (2007) The transtheoretical model of intentional behaviour change. *Drugs and Alcohol Today,* 7 (1): 29–32.

Dixon, A (2008) *Motivation and Confidence: What Does It Take to Change Behaviour?* London: King's Fund.

DiZazzo-Miller, R, Samuel, PS, Barnas, JM and Welker, KM (2014) Addressing everyday challenges: feasibility of a family caregiver training program for people with dementia. *American Journal of Occupational Therapy*, 68 (2): 212–20.

Douglas-Dunbar, M and Gardiner, P (2007) Support for carers of people with dementia during hospital admission. *Nursing Older People*, 19 (8): 27–30.

Drennan, V and Goodman, C (2014) *Oxford Handbook of Primary Care and Community Nursing*, 2nd edn. Oxford: Oxford University Press.

Driscoll, J (1994) Reflective practice for practice. *Senior Nurse*, 14 (1): 47–50.

Duerden, M, Avery, T and Payne, R (2013) *Polypharmacy and Medicines Optimisation: Making It Safe and Sound*. London: The King's Fund.

Emerson, E and Baines, S (2010) *Health Inequalities and People with Learning Disabilities in the UK: Improving Health and Lives 2010*. [Online] Available from: www.improvinghealthandlives.org.uk/uploads/doc/vid_7479_IHaL2010–3HealthInequality2010.pdf [Accessed: 10/05/15].

Endacott, R, Jevon, P and Cooper, S (eds) (2009) *Clinical Nursing Skills: Core and Advanced*. Oxford: Oxford University Press.

European Network on Patient Empowerment (2012) *Patient Empowerment – Living with Chronic Disease: A series of short discussion topics on different aspects of self-management and patient empowerment for the 1st European Conference on Patient Empowerment*. The First European Conference on Patient Empowerment. Copenhagen, Denmark, 11–12 April 2012. [Online] Available from: www.enope.eu/media/14615/a_series_of_short_discussion_topics_on_different.pdf [Accessed: 05/03/15].

Excellence Gateway (2015) *Skilled for Health*. [Online] Available from: http://rwp.excellencegateway.org.uk/Embedded%20Learning/Skilled%20for%20Health [Accessed: 05/03/15].

Felce, D, Baxter, H, Lowe, K, Dunstan, F, Houston, H, Jones, G, Felce, J and Kerr, M (2008) The impact of repeated health checks for adults with learning disabilities. *Journal of Applied Research in Intellectual Disabilities*. Journal Compilation. Oxford: Blackwell Publishing.

Flynn, R and Mulcahy, H (2013) Early-onset dementia: the impact on family care-givers. *British Journal of Community Nursing*, 18 (12): 598–606.

Gardner, H (1983; 1993) *Frames of Mind: The Multiple Intelligences*. New York: Basic Books. (Second edition was published in Britain by Fontana Press.)

Gardner, H (1999) *Intelligence Reframed: Multiple Intelligences for the 21st Century*. New York: Basic Books.

General Medical Council (2013a) *End of Life Care: Advance Care Planning*. [Online] Available from: www.gmc-uk.org/guidance/ethical_guidance/end_of_life_advance_care_planning.asp [Accessed: 20/05/15].

General Medical Council (2013b) *Good Medical Practice*. [Online] Available from: www.gmc-uk.org/guidance/good_medical_practice.asp [Accessed: 20/05/15].

Gibson, G, Newton, L, Pritchard, G, Finch, T, Brittain, K and Robinson, L (2014) The provision of assistive technology services for people with dementia. *Dementia*, 2014: 1–21.

Gold Standards Framework (2015) *Advance Care Planning*. [Online] Available from: www.goldstandardsframework.org.uk/advance-care-planning [Accessed: 20/05/15].

Gomes, B, Calanzini, N, Gysels, M, Hall, S and Higginson, J (2013) Heterogeneity and changes in preferences for dying at home: a systematic review. *BNC Palliative Care*, 12 (7).

Haddad, M (2010) Caring for patients with long-term conditions and depression. *Nursing Standard*, 24 (24): 40–9.

Heath, H, Sturdy, D and Wilcock, G (2010) *Improving Quality of Care for People with Dementia in General Hospitals*. London: RCN Publishing.

Hibbard, JH, Mahoney, ER, Stockard, J and Tusler, M (2005) Development and testing of a short form of the patient activation measure. *Journal of Health Services Research*, 40 (6p1): 1918–30.

Hickin, S, Renshaw, J, Williams, R, Horton-Szar, D and Usamani, OS (2013) *Crash Course: Respiratory System*, 4th edn. Edinburgh: Mosby Elsevier.

Higginson, IJ, Sarmento, VP, Calanzani, N, Benalia, H and Gomes, B (2013) Dying at home – is it better: a narrative appraisal of the state of the science. *Palliative Medicine*, 27 (10): 918–24.

House of Commons Health Committee (2009) *Health Inequalities: Third Report of Session 2008–2009*. London: The Stationery Office.

Huang, SL, Li, CM, Yang, CY and Chen, JJJ (2009) Application of reminiscence treatment on older people with dementia: a case study in Pingtung, Taiwan. *Journal of Nursing Research*, 17 (2): 112–18.

Janata, P (2012) Effects of widespread and frequent personalised music programming on agitation and depression in assisted living facility residents with Alzheimer-type dementia. *Music and Medicine*, 4 (1): 8–15.

Kaufman, G (2014) Polypharmacy, medicines optimisation and concordance. *Nurse Prescribing*, 12 (4): 197–201.

Kaye, P (1996) *Breaking Bad News (Pocket Book)*. Northampton: EPL Publications.

Keogh, Professor Sir Bruce (2013) *Review into the Quality of Care and Treatment Provided by 14 Hospital Trusts in England: Overview Report*. [Online] Available from: www.nhs.uk/NHSEngland/bruce-keogh-review/Documents/outcomes/keogh-review-final-report.pdf [Accessed: 15/01/15].

Kickbusch, IS (2001) Health literacy: addressing the health and education divide. *Health Promotion International*, 16 (3): 289–97.

Kivimäki, M, Hammer, M, Batty, GD, Geddes, JR, Tabak, AG, Pentti, A, Virtanen, M and Vahtera, J (2010) Antidepressant medication use, weight gain, and risk of type 2 diabetes. *Diabetes Care*, 33 (12): 2611–16. [Online] Available from: http://care.diabetesjournals.org/content/33/12/2611.full.pdf+html [Accessed: 15/01/15].

Knai, C (2009) What is public health? In: Thornbory, G (ed.) (2009) *Pubic Health Nursing: A Textbook for Health Visitors, School Nurses and Occupational Health Nurses*. Oxford: Blackwell Publishing, pp. 1–16.

Knight, J (2009) Songs for learning. *Nursing Standard*, 23 (43): 22–3.

Kübler-Ross, E (2009) *On Death and Dying: What the Dying Have to Teach Doctors, Nurses, Clergy and Their Own Family*, 40th Anniversary edn. Abingdon: Routledge.

Kübler-Ross, E and Kessler, D (2005) *On Grief and Grieving: Finding the Meaning of Grief Through the Five Stages of Loss*. London: Simon Schuster.

Lalkhen, AG, Bedrod, JP and Dwuer, AD (2012) Pain associated with multiple sclerosis: epidemiology, classification and management. *British Journal of Neuroscience Nursing*, 8 (5): 267–74.

Lewis, V, Bauer, M, Winbolt, M, Chenco, C and Hanley, F (2015) A study of the effectiveness of MP3 players to support family carers of people living with dementia at home. *International Psychogeriatrics*, 27 (3): 471–9.

Lindsey, M (2002) Comprehensive health care services for people with learning disabilities. *Advances in Psychiatric Treatment*, 8: 138–47.

Lorig, K, Holman, H, Sobel, D, Laurent, D, Gonzales, V and Minor, M (2006) *Living a Healthy Life with Chronic Conditions: Self-Management of Heart Disease, Arthritis, Diabetes, Asthma, Bronchitis, Emphysema and Others*. Boulder: Bull Publishing Company.

Lorig, K, Laurent, DD, Plant, K, Krishnan, E and Ritter, PL (2014) The components of action planning and their association with behaviour and health outcomes. *Chronic Illness*, 10 (1): 50–9.

McAllister, M, Dunn, G, Payne, K, Davies, L and Todd, C (2012) Patient empowerment: the need to consider it as a measurable patient-reported outcome for chronic conditions. *BMC Health Services Research*, 12: 157–64.

McDonald, C (2014) *Patients in Control: Why People with Long-Term Conditions Must be Empowered*. London: Institute for Public Policy Research.

McGrath, A and Yeowart, C (2009) *Rights of Passage: Supporting Disabled Young People Through the Transition to Adulthood*. London: New Philanthropy Capital.

McKenna, J (2007) Emotional intelligence training in adjustment to physical disability and illness. *International Journal of Therapy and Rehabilitation*, 14 (12): 551–6.

Marmot, M (2010) *Fair Society: Healthy Lives (The Marmot Review)*. London: The Marmot Review.

Mason, P (2008) Motivational interviewing. *Practice Nurse*, 35 (3).

Mental Capacity Act (2015) [Online] Available from: www.legislation.gov.uk/ukpga/2005/9/contents [Accessed: 20/05/15].

Mezuk, B, Eaton, WW, Albrecht, S and Golden, SH (2008) Depression and type 2 diabetes over the lifespan: a meta analysis. *Diabetes Care*, 31 (12): 2383–90.

Middleton, S, Barnett, J and Reeves, D (2001) *What Is an Integrated Care Pathway?* [Online] Available from: www.medicine.ox.ac.uk/bandolier/painres/download/whatis/What_is_an_ICP.pdf [Accessed: 14/05/15].

Morse, JM (1991) Negotiating commitment and involvement in the nurse–patient relationship. *Journal of Advanced Nursing*, 16 (4): 455–68. First published online July 2007 DOI: 10.1111/j.1365–2648.1991.tb03436.x.

Moskowitz, JT, Hult, JR, Bussolari, C and Acree, M (2009) What works in coping with HIV? A meta-analysis with implications for coping with serious illness. *Psychological Bulletin*, 135 (1): 121–41.

Munday, D, Petrova, M and Dale, J (2009) Exploring preferences for place of death with terminally ill patients: qualitative study of experiences of general practitioners and community nurses in England. *British Medical Journal*, 339: b2391.

Muralitharan, M and Peate, I (2013) *Fundamentals of Applied Pathophysiology: An Essential Guide for Nursing and Healthcare Students*. Singapore: Wiley-Blackwell.

Murphy, J and Oliver, T (2013) The use of Talking Mats to support people with dementia and their carers to make decisions together. *Health and Social Care in the Community*, 21 (2): 171–80.

Naidoo, J and Wills, J (2009) *Foundations for Health Promotion (Public Health and Health Promotion*, 3rd edn). China: Bailliere Tindall, Elsevier.

Narayanan, V, Bista, B and Koshy, C (2010) 'BREAKS' protocol for breaking bad news. *Indian Journal of Palliative Care*, 16 (2): 61–5.

National Advisory Group on the Safety of Patients in England (2013) *A Promise to Learn – A Commitment to Act: Improving the Safety of Patients in England*. [Online] Available from: www.gov.uk/government/uploads/system/uploads/attachment_data/file/226703/Berwick_Report.pdf [Accessed: 14/05/15].

National Centre for Palliative Care (2008) *Advance Care Planning: A Guide for Health and Social Care Staff*. Leicester: End of Life Care Programme.

National Collaborating Centre for Mental Health (2007) *Dementia: A NICE-SCIE Guideline on Supporting People with Dementia and Their Carers in Health and Social Care.* Leicester and London: The British Psychological Society and The Royal College of Psychiatrists.

National Health Service Improving Quality (2010) *Holistic Common Assessment of Supporting and Palliative Care Needs for Adults Requiring End of Life Care.* London: NHS Improving Quality.

National Institute for Health and Care Excellence (2005) *Medicines Optimisation: The Safe and Effective Use of Medicines to Enable the Best Possible Outcome.* [Online] Available from: www.nice.org.uk/guidance/NG5/chapter/Introduction [Accessed: 14/05/15].

National Institute for Health and Clinical Excellence (2009a) *Depression in Adults with a Chronic Physical Health Problem: Treatment and Management.* London: NICE.

National Institute for Health and Clinical Excellence (2009b) *Depression: The Treatment and Management of Depression in Adults (partial update of NICE Guideline 23).* London: NICE.

National Institute for Health and Care Excellence (2009c) *Medicines Adherence: Involving Patients in Decisions about Prescribed Medicines and Supporting Adherence.* [Online] Available from: www.nice.org.uk/guidance/cg76/chapter/Introduction#ftn.footnote_1 [Accessed: 14/05/15].

Nawate, Y, Kaneko, F, Hanaoka, H and Okamura, H (2008) Efficacy of group reminiscence therapy for elderly dementia patients residing at home: a preliminary report. *Physical and Occupational Therapy in Geriatrics,* 26 (3): 57–68.

NHS Employers (2009) *Quality and Outcomes Framework Guidance for GMS Contract 2009/10: Delivering Investment in General Practice.* England, NHS Employers.

NHS Employers (2014) *2014/15 General Medical Services (GMS) Contract Quality and Outcomes Framework (QOF): Guidance for GMS Contract 2014/15.* [Online] Available from: www.nhsemployers.org/~/media/Employers/Documents/Primary%20care%20contracts/QOF/2014–15/2014–15%20General%20Medical%20Services%20contract%20-%20%20Quality%20and%20Outcomes%20Framework%20Guidance.pdf [Accessed: 07/06/15].

NHS England (2014) *Five Year Forward View.* [Online] Available from: www.england.nhs.uk/wp-content/uploads/2014/10/5yfv-web.pdf [Accessed: 07/06/15].

NHS Institute for Innovation and Improvement (2010) *High Impact Actions for Nursing and Midwifery: The Essential Collection.* [Online] Available from: www.institute.nhs.uk/building_capability/general/aims [Accessed: 16/05/15].

NHS Modernisation Agency and Skills for Health (2005) *Case Management Competencies Framework.* London: Department of Health.

NHS Quality Improvement Scotland (2007) *Standards for Integrated Care Pathways for Mental Health.* Edinburgh: NHS Quality Improvement Scotland.

NHS Scotland (2010) *Long Term Conditions Collaborative: Improving Care Pathways.* [Online] Available from: www.scotland.gov.uk/Resource/Doc/309257/0097421.pdf [Accessed: 07/06/15].

Nicholson, A, Kuper, H and Hemingway, H (2006) Depression as an aetiologic and prognostic factor in coronary heart disease: a meta-analysis of 6362 events among 146 538 participants in 54 observational studies. *European Heart Journal,* 27 (23): 2763–74.

Nursing and Midwifery Council (2010) *Standards for Pre-Registration Nursing Education.* London: NMC.

Nursing and Midwifery Council (2015) *The Code: Professional Standards of Practice and Behaviour for Nurses and Midwives.* London: Nursing and Midwifery Council.

Nutbeam, D (1999) Health Promotion Glossary. *Health Promotion International,* 13 (4): 349–64.

Nutbeam, D (2000) Health literacy as a public health goal: a challenge for contemporary health education and communication strategies into the 21st century. *Health Promotion International,* 15 (3): 259–67.

Office for National Statistics (2011) *National Population Projections, 2010-Based Statistical Bulletin.* [Online] Available from: www.ons.gov.uk/ons/dcp171778_235886.pdf [Accessed: 07/06/15].

Office for National Statistics (2014a) *8 Facts about Life Expectancy and the 90 and Over Population.* [Online] Available from: www.ons.gov.uk/ons/rel/lifetables/national-life-tables/2010–2012/sty-facts-about-le.html [Accessed: 13/01/15].

Office for National Statistics (2014b) *Life Expectancy at Birth and at Age 65 by Local Area in the United Kingdom, 2006–08 to 2010–12.* [Online] Available from: http://ons.gov.uk/ons/dcp171778_360047.pdf [Accessed: 07/06/15].

Offredy, M, Bunn, F and Morgan, J (2009) Case management in long term conditions: an inconsistent journey? *British Journal of Community Nursing,* 14 (6): 252–7.

Okomura, Y, Tanimukai, S and Asada, T (2008) Effects of short-term reminiscence therapy on elderly with dementia: a comparison with everyday conversation approaches. *Psychogeriatrics,* 8: 124–33.

Orem, DE (1980) *Nursing: Concepts of Practice.* New York: McGraw Hill.

Papastravrou, E, Kalokerniou, A, Papacostas, SS, Tsangari, H and Sourtzi, P (2007) Caring for a relative with dementia: family caregiver burden. *Journal of Advanced Nursing: Original Research.* Journal Compilation. Oxford: Blackwell Publishing.

Phillips, J (2009) Improving access to self-management services. *British Journal of Neuroscience Nursing,* 5 (11): 524–5.

Poppe, C, Crombez, G, Hanoulle, I, Vogelaers, D and Petrovic, M (2013) Improving quality of life in patients with chronic kidney disease. *Nephrology Dialysis Transplantation,* 28 (1): 116–21.

Porth, CM and Matfin, G (2010) *Essentials of Pathophysiology: Concepts of Altered Health Status (International Edition).* Wolters Kluwer Health/Lippincott: Williams and Wilkins.

Randall, S, Daly, G, Thunhurst, C, Mills, N, Guest, DA and Barker, A (2014) Case management of individuals with long-term conditions by community matrons: report of qualitative findings of a mixed method evaluation. *Primary Healthcare Research,* 15: 26–37.

Raphael, D, Steinmetz, B, Renwick, R, Rootman, I, Brown, I, Sehdev, H, Phillips, S and Smith, T (1999) The Community Quality of Life Project: a health promotion approach to understanding communities. *Health Promotion International,* 14 (3): 197–210.

RCN (2012) *RCN Fact Sheet: Nurse Prescribing in the UK.* [Online] Available from: www.rcn.org.uk/__data/assets/pdf_file/0008/443627/Nurse_Prescribing_in_the_UK_-_RCN_Factsheet.pdf [Accessed: 07/06/15].

Rhudy, L, Holland, D and Bowels, K (2009) Illuminating hospital discharge planning: staff nurse decision making. *Applied Nursing Research,* 23: 198–206.

Rogers, CR (1967) *On Becoming a Person: A Therapist's View of Psychotherapy.* London: Constable.

Roper, N, Logan, WW and Tierney, AJ (2000) *Roper-Logan-Tierney Model of Nursing: The Activities of Daily Living Model.* Edinburgh: Churchill Livingstone.

Rosness, TA, Mjorud, M and Engedal, K (2011) Quality of life and depression in carers of patients with early onset dementia. *Aging and Mental Health,* 15 (3): 299–306.

Royal College of General Practitioners (2008) *Prognostic Indicator Guidance.* [Online] Available at: www. goldstandardsframework.org.uk/cd-content/uploads/files/General%20Files/Prognostic%20Indicator %20Guidance%20October%202011.pdf [Accessed: 07/06/15].

Royal College of General Practitioners (2013) *Matters of Life and Death: Helping People to Live Well Until They Die.* London: Royal College of General Practitioners.

Royal College of Nursing (2003) *Defining Nursing: Nursing is . . .* London: Royal College of Nursing.

Royal College of Physicians (2010) *Passive Smoking and Children: A Report by the Tobacco Advisory Group of the Royal College of Physicians.* London: Royal College of Physicians.

Royal Commission on Long Term Care (1999) *With Respect to Old Age: Long Term Care – Rights and Responsibilities.* London: The Stationery Office.

Salovey, P and Mayer, JD (1990) *Emotional Intelligence.* [Online] Available from: www.unh.edu/emotional_ intelligence/EIAssets/EmotionalIntelligenceProper? [Accessed: 07/06/15].

Saunders, C (1994) The medicalization of death. *European Journal of Cancer Care (Engl),* Dec. 3 (4): 148.

Scottish Intercollegiate Guidelines Network (2014) *SIGN 141 – British Guideline on the Management of Asthma.* [Online] Available from: www.brit-thoracic.org.uk/document-library/clinical-information/asthma/bts- sign-asthma-guideline–2014 [Accessed: 13/05/15].

Shepperd, S, Lannin, NA, Clemson, LM, McCluskey, A, Cameron, ID and Barras, SL (2013) *Discharge Planning from Hospital to Home (Review).* [Online] Available from: http://onlinelibrary.wiley.com/doi/ 10.1002/14651858.CD000313.pub4/pdf [Accessed: 16/05/15].

Silva, AL, Teixeira, HJ, Texeira, MJC and Freitas, S (2013) The needs of informal caregivers of elderly peo- ple living at home: an integrative review. *Scandinavian Journal of Caring Science,* 27 (4): 792–803.

Simon, C, Everitt, H, van Dorp, F and Burkes, M (2014) *Oxford Handbook of General Practice,* 4th edn. Oxford: Oxford University Press.

Smith, MK (1997, 2002) Paulo Freire and informal education. *The Encyclopaedia of Informal Education.* [Online] Available from: www.infed.org/thinkers/et-freir.htm [Accessed: 07/06/2015].

Smith, P (1992) *The Emotional Labour of Nursing: How Nurses Care.* Basingstoke: Macmillan Press.

Stirling, C, Andrews, S, Croft, T, Vickers, J, Turner, P and Robinson, A (2010) Measuring dementia carers' unmet need for services: an exploratory mixed method study. *Health Services Research,* 10: 122.

Sutherland, D and Hayter, M (2009) Structured review: evaluating the effectiveness of nurse case man- agers in improving health outcomes for three major chronic diseases. *Journal of Clinical Nursing,* 18 (21): 2978–92.

Sykes, S, Wills, J, Rowlands, G and Popple, K (2013) Understanding critical health literacy: a concept analysis. *BMC Public Health,* 13: 150.

Taverner, T (2014) Neuropathic pain: an overview. *British Journal of Neuroscience Nursing,* 10 (3): 116–23.

Tebes, JK, Irish, JT, Puglisi-Vasquez, MJ and Perkins, DV (2004) Cognitive transformation as a marker of resilience. *Substance Use and Misuse,* 39: 769–88.

Telford, K, Kralik, D and Koch, T (2006) Acceptance and denial: implications for people adapting to chronic illness: a literature review. *Journal of Advanced Nursing,* 55 (4): 457–64.

The Cavendish Review (2013) *An Independent Review into Healthcare Assistants and Support Workers in the NHS and Social Care Settings.* [Online] Available from: www.gov.uk/government/uploads/system/uploads/ attachment_data/file/236212/Cavendish_Review.pdf [Accessed: 07/06/15].

References

The Mid Staffordshire NHS Foundation Trust Public Inquiry (2013) *Report of the Mid Staffordshire NHS Foundation Trust Public Inquiry: Executive Summary.* London: The Stationery Office.

Thomas, K (2003) *Caring for the Dying at Home: Companions on the Journey.* Abingdon: Radcliffe Medical Press.

Toofany, S (2006) Patient empowerment: myth or reality? *Nursing Management* 13 (6): 18–22.

Tuffrey-Wijne, I (2012) A new model for breaking bad news to people with intellectual disabilities. *Palliative Medicine*, 27 (1): 5–12.

Van Gils, PF, Tariq, L, Verschuuren, M and van der Berg, M (2010) Cost effectiveness research on preventative interventions: a survey of the publications in 2008. *European Journal of Public Health*, 21 (2): 260–4.

Wales Audit Office (2014) *The Management of Chronic Conditions in Wales: An Update.* [Online] Available from: www.wao.gov.uk/system/files/publications/The%20Management%20of%20Chronic%20Conditions%20in%20Wales%20-%20An%20Update.pdf [Accessed: 07/06/15].

Waller, S (2012) Redesigning wards to support people with dementia in hospital. *Nursing Older People*, 24 (2): 16–21.

Wilmot, J (2002) Palliative care of non-malignant conditions. In: Charlton, R (ed.) *Primary Palliative Care: Dying Death and Bereavement in the Community.* Abingdon: Radcliffe Medical Press.

World Health Organization (1997) *WHOQOL: Measuring Quality of Life.* Geneva: WHO.

World Health Organization (1998) *Health Promotion Glossary.* Geneva: World Health Organization.

World Health Organization (2002) *National Cancer Control Programmes: Policies and Managerial Guidelines.* Geneva: World Health Organization.

World Health Organization (2009) *Milestones in Health Promotion: Statements from Global Conferences.* Geneva: World Health Organization.

World Health Organization (2010) *The Determinants of Health.* [Online] Available from: www.who.int/hia/evidence/doh/en [Accessed: 07/06/15].

World Health Organization (2013) *Noncommunicable Diseases.* [Online] Available from: www.who.int/mediacentre/factsheets/fs355/en/ [Accessed: 07/06/15].

Yura, H and Walsh, MB (1973) *The Nursing Process: Assessing, Planning, Implementing, Evaluating.* New York: Appleton Century Crofts.

Index

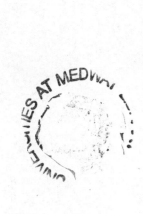